Power, Freedom and Flow

Your Journey to Health and Happiness

By David-Dorian Ross

©Copyright 2003
Wellness Evolution Press   San Jose, CA.

Coypright ©2003 by David-Dorian Ross. Printed and bound in the United States of America. All rights reserved. No part of this book may be reproduced or transmitted in any form or by any means, electronic or mechanical, including photocopying, recording, or by an information storage and retrieval system – except by a reviewer who may quote brief passages in a review to be printed in a magazine or newspaper – without permission is writing from the publisher. For information, contact The Wellness Evolution Press, 540 N. Santa Cruz Avenue, Suite 216, Los Gatos, CA 95030, 408-499-6101.

This book contains information gathered from many sources. It is published as general reference and not as a substitute for independent verification by users when circumstances warrant. It is sold with the understanding that neither the author nor the publisher is engaged in any legal, medical or psychological advice. The publisher and author disclaim any personal liability, either directly or indirectly, for advice or information presented within. Although the author and publisher have used care and diligence in the preparation, and made every effort to ensure the accuracy and completeness of information contained in this book, we assume no responsibility for errors, inaccuracies, omissions or any inconsistencies herein. Any slights of people, places, books or organizations are unintentional.

First printing 2003

Ross, David-Dorian
    Power, Freedom and Flow: Your Journey to Health and Happiness / David-Dorian Ross
    Includes bibliographical references, charts and illustrations.
    ISBN (trade paper)
    1. Books – United States – Health   I. Ross, David-Dorian 1957 –
    II. Title

ALSO BY DAVID-DORIAN ROSS

Books

    The T'ai Chi Companion Workbook, Vol. 1 (Yang Style Short Form)

    The Mind/Body Personal Trainer: A Handbook for Holistic Practice

    Exercising the Soul: How T'ai Chi Nurtures the BodyMind (Coming in 2004)

Video/DVD

    T'ai Chi with David-Dorian Ross

    Flow Motion: The Simplified T'ai Chi Workout

    A.M. Chi for Beginners

    Energy Chi for Beginners

    Upper Body Chi for Beginners

    Lower Body Chi for Beginners

Acknowledgements

There are so many of you I wish to thank that there are not enough pages in any book to list your names and honor you. You have either directly or indirectly influenced my thoughts, provided support and inspiration, and encouraged me to continue. I continue to add to the list every day, but just a very small roll would have to include the following: my mother, Nona Ross; Mary Aldridge; Grandmaster Doc-Fai Wong; C.J. Willson; Bob Adams, Ron Kramer and Myron Wong; Ralph LaForge, Pamela Peeke, Peter and Kathie Davis and Patti McCord; Beth Rothenberg; Nora Anderson; Tom Stone; David Lepp; Leslie Flowers; Lorna, Shannon and Lance Coffel and all my family at River's Edge; and Michelle Pate – lover, muse, inspiration and best girl. I remember you all in my prayers every day for your teaching, your friendship and your faith in me.

I also want to thank every one of my clients and students (another long list, but I hope you know who you are); Landmark Education; Coachville.com; Ken Wilber (for being a huge source of inspiration); Gaiam International; Hawaii Public Television; and both Starbucks and Borders Books for unknowingly supplying creative workspace.

HOW TO CONTACT THE AUTHOR

Professional speaker, author and expert Wellness Coach David-Dorian Ross has been delighting and informing audiences in fitness, wellness and health organizations for more than two decades. David-Dorian has also spoken to business leaders, government groups, medical professionals, public educators and service organizations around the world. He speaks about the holistic, mind/body/Spirit approach to health and happiness in a way that makes it easy for anyone to understand, embrace and employ in their own lives. To discuss hiring him for your next conference, fund-raiser or special event, contact:

David-Dorian Ross

The Wellness Evolution

POB 216 540 N. Santa Cruz Ave. Los Gatos, CA 95030

Phone: 408-499-6101; email: drtaichi@aol.com

Web: www.thewellnessevolution.com

WANT TO KNOW MORE ABOUT THE WELLNESS EVOLUTION?

The Wellness Evolution is an online, global community of holistic health practitioners as well as non-professionals simply interested in an holistic approach to health and happiness. We provide training, education and certification opportunities, professional resources (many of them at no cost), information sharing and links to other providers. The Wellness Evolution is a forum for having a new conversation about what is possible in the world of fitness, wellness and health. For more information, visit our website at www.thewellnessevolution.com.

<u>Dedication</u>

To my father, Dr. Dorian M. Ross.
You're still my hero.
And to my son, Zachery.

I miss you both.

Table of Contents

ACKNOWLEDGEMENTS 5
THE GREATEST DOCTOR IN THE WORLD 14
CHAPTER I: REVELATION 16
   A World Without Suffering 17
   There is nothing wrong with you 21
   Physical Culture 26
   What's Going On? 29
   Two Differing Paradigms 32
      The Conventional Paradigm 34
      The Holistic Paradigm 41
   Power, Freedom and Flow 49
   Masks of the BodyMind 51
   Revelation 53
      Exercise 55
   A Final Thought 56
CHAPTER II: THE FIVE SEASONS OF THE BODYMIND 58
   Who Are You? 59
   Recognizing Mind/Body Types 62
   Personality and Temperament 63
   The History of Typing 67
   The 5 Seasons of the BodyMind 71
      Spring - The Lion 72
      Summer - The Horse 75
      Indian Summer - The Bear 80
      Autumn – The Fox 83
      Winter – The Ox 86
      Take the Test -- Discover your own BodyMind Season ... 89
   A Final Thought 92
CHAPTER III: ELEMENTS 95
   Happiness 97
      Balance 100
      The Wellness Triangle 102
      Integrity, Compassion and Synergy 103
      Sensation/Perception Cycle 105
      Spontaneous Healing 107
   Unmasking the BodyMind 108
      The Six Universal Compensations 114
         Heaviness 114
         Lightness 116
         Breaking 116
         Stiffness 117
         Misdirection 118

    Monotony 118
    A Final Thought.. *120*
DESIDERATUM #1: FITNESS, WELLNESS & HEALTH 126
    Fitness, Wellness and Health... *127*
        Fitness.. 128
        Wellness 128
        Health 129
    Fitness *130*
        Is Fitness for You?... 130
        The Training Effect 131
        The Beauty of Fitness 132
    Wellness.. *133*
        What's the Difference? 135
    Health *138*
DESIDERATUM #2: THE THREE CONTINUA 142
    Three Continua (Exercise, Diet, Relaxation) *143*
    Design 101... *144*
    The Workout Continuum.. *146*
        Conventional Exercise... 146
        Modern Mind/Body Exercise 147
        Classical Mind/Body Exercise.. 148
    The Diet Continuum *150*
    The Relaxation Continuum *153*
CHAPTER IV: KINESIOLOGY 158
    The Science of Motion *159*
    A Body Out of Balance *164*
    Compensations and Muscle Imbalances..................................... *165*
    Exercise *167*
    A Glossary of Symptoms.. *169*
    A Final Thought.. *172*
CHAPTER V: CONVERSATIONS OF THE BODY 176
    The Body as Metaphor... *177*
    The Discovery Process *186*
    Looking in the Mirror.. *188*
    Unmasking the BodyMind *189*
    Case Study: Finding Freedom... *190*
    A Final Thought.. *194*
CHAPTER VI: A RECIPE FOR TRANSFORMATION 198
    Four Phases of Transformation.. *202*
    Whipping Up Your Holistic Program.. *204*
        Step One: Look in the Mirror 204
            The 5-Season BodyMind Type Test................................205
            The Wellness Index Survey 206
            Simple Postural Assessment..207

    Step Two: Distinguish Your Patterns.. 208
        Review the 6 Universal Compensations Chart............................ 208
        Review the Continua... 209
        The Balancing Acts.. 210
    Step Three: Mix your choices according to your BodyMind Season, and serve. 212
        Sample Six-Week Programs -- Phase One: Discovery. 214
  A Final Thought 222
GENESIS.. 226
  Healing the Soul of the World.. 227
  Namaste... 238

The Greatest Doctor in the World
(An Holistic Parable)

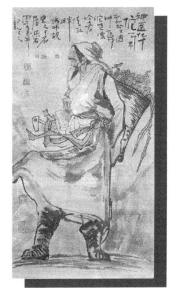

Once upon a time, in the days when China was ruled by an emperor, there lived a doctor who was so wise that he could cure any illness. All around his village, the people knew they could go to him with any disease, or injury, or disfigurement, and the doctor would be able to heal them. No condition was too severe for the doctor's special combination of herbs and acupuncture.

As the doctor's fame spread far and wide, the common people began to call him, "The Greatest Doctor in the World." And before too long, word of this incredible healer reached the ears of the Emperor himself.

"We must invite him to our court," said the Emperor, "for if he is the greatest doctor in the world, we must have him for our royal physician."

When the doctor arrived at the Emperor's court, he bowed low to the ground.

"What an honor to be summoned before your Imperial Majesty," said the doctor. "But I'm not quite sure why I am here."

"Well," said the Emperor, "we heard you were the greatest doctor in the world. Of course we wanted to meet you."

The doctor nodded his head, as if he finally understood something that had been puzzling him. "You have given me great face for complimenting me so. But actually I am not the *greatest* doctor in the world. I am very good, but there is one who is greater: my brother."

The Emperor was dumbfounded. "Your brother?" he exclaimed. "How is it that we have never heard of *him?*"

"Well you see," began the doctor, "all the people who come to me are already sick and suffering, so when I cure them of course they rejoice loudly and tell all their friends and family about me. But my wise brother has taught all the people in his village how to exercise like the animals of the forest, how to eat only the fresh foods of the land, and how to stay happy in their hearts. He has taught everyone in his village how to *stay healthy*. No one in his village ever gets sick, and so no one ever hears about them having to get well. But this is precisely why *he* is truly the greatest doctor in the world."

Chapter I: Revelation

Think of every chapter of this book as a present to be unwrapped. The gift of the first chapter, Revelation, is *clarity*. This chapter illustrates our current paradigm of what it means to be fit, well and healthy -- and then explains in detail an alternative to that paradigm. Open this gift, and I hope to hear you say, "I now have a new way of thinking about my life and my health."

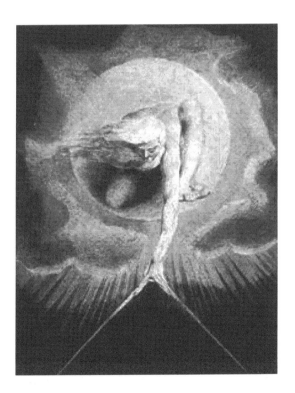

A World Without Suffering

Imagine a world in which everyone who wanted to could live to be 100 years old, free from chronic pain, injury or disease. All the people in such a world would be emotionally fulfilled and each one able to experience the joy of unrestricted movement in work and play. Think of the peace and freedom we could each individually enjoy in a world liberated from the experience of painful aging or untimely death.

What do you think it would it take to live in a world in which the money now spent on hospitals, acute medical care and nursing for the elderly was not needed, and was allocated instead to educating the young, feeding the hungry and cleaning up our environment? What would it be like to live in a world that minimized the physical suffering that now aggravates our normal human fears and insecurities?

When I dream of the future, I see a world freed from the torments of war, hatred, poverty, hunger, prejudice and violence. At the same time, I see that the problems that affect us globally are not more important than – indeed are not separate from – the challenges that we face daily in our own families and communities. How can we be expected to be kind, loving and patient when we are caught up in our own suffering?

Suffering, just to be clear, is not the same thing as *pain*. Pain is something we feel, a human experience just as natural as happiness or curiosity. Suffering, on the other hand, is how we choose to feel *about* our pain. Imagine freedom from suffering as learning to let go of the stories we make up to explain away our hurts and fears. Our emancipation begins when we consider that all suffering has the same source: the disconnection from self. Our experience of suffering begins the moment when – somewhere, somehow – we cut ourselves off from who we are. From that instant on, we are walking around feeling less than whole, and our world feels like something is missing, or like something is wrong.

Consider instead a Holistic approach to life. Imagine learning how to flow through life joyfully aware of the interweaving of body, mind, emotions and Spirit within us – and intimately connected as well to the people, ideas and events in our lives. Suffering would fade away, like mist warmed by the rising sun and scattered by the breeze. In the following pages, I want to engage you in a conversation about what is possible in the realm of your health and happiness.

This book has four simple goals:

1) To introduce you to a new holistic way of looking at your life and your health;

2) To give you the power to choose between the Holistic approach or the Conventional approach (by explaining the details and distinctions of each);

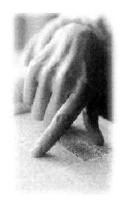

3) To help you discover your BodyMind type – the unique combination of psychological and physiological characteristics that make you who you are; and

4) To offer you a set of basic tools that will help you begin your journey to health and happiness.

All too often our physical bodies are the first place we feel pain and suffering. It is, therefore, one of the first places we disconnect from ourselves. We start out with a complaint (I'm too fat). The complaint turns into a story, a subconscious explanation about what's "wrong" (being fat is ugly, nobody likes fat people, and I don't feel loveable when I look this way). The story becomes a reason to disconnect, and puts us in conflict with ourselves (I hate my body, but I'll feel better when I lose some weight).

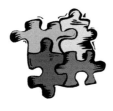

The Holistic approach to life is fundamentally about being connected and whole. More accurately, you could say that the Holistic approach is about having an *experience* of being connected and whole. As you will see, we can never really be less than whole, although we can *feel* incomplete. When we talk about disconnection or dissociation, we are actually talking about being in a state of self-denial, consciously or unconsciously trying to escape from whom we authentically are.

Yet magically, the more we honor and connect to our authentic selves – the inherently perfect interwoven threads of body, mind, emotion and Spirit – the *less* we suffer. In short, the Holistic approach is a reflection of the most basic purpose of human life: to treat our time on earth as a voyage of Self-discovery, embracing moment by moment anything and everything that will educe, evoke and evolve the experience of our authentic self. That experience is our ticket to the future I dream about, a world in which we understand that we only suffer if we choose to suffer. And what better place to begin that voyage to discover our authentic identity than in the way we relate to our material selves?

> *"From the beginning Western cultures have seemed almost driven to perfect the world, to make it better."* -- John Bradshaw

There is *nothing* wrong with you.

The primary difference between the Holistic approach and the Conventional approach is that the Conventional, Western approach to fitness, wellness and health begins with the assumption that *something is wrong with you* that needs to be fixed or improved. The Holistic approach, on the other hand, begins with the assumption that you are already perfect, and anything that doesn't look or feel perfect is merely your perfection *concealed*.

Just this morning I had an opportunity to work with a young woman who has been suffering from severe lower back pain and sciatica – pain that started in her back and radiated all the way down her leg. What struck me initially was that she was so young – early 20's – and she had already had surgery to relieve the pressure on her sciatic nerve from bulging discs in her lower back. Her condition doesn't usually show up in someone her age. We did some basic muscle tests, and I asked her some questions about what her doctors had done, and what they had told her.

Finally, when I had satisfied myself that I had a fairly complete picture of her condition, I gave her some suggestions about exercise to strengthen the muscles that support her back, and I gave her a quick outline of the cycle of pain, postural distortion and muscle atrophy. And then I told her what I tell all my clients. "Here's the thing, Sophie. There is nothing wrong with you. You've been in pain, and when that goes on for an extended period we start to feel like we're broken and not OK. But you *are* OK, and you are *not* broken. Remember that built into your physical and Spiritual DNA is all the information your body needs to heal itself completely. All we need to find is the right access to let that happen."

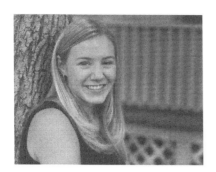

I could see her eyes begin to water. "Thank you," she said. "That's the first time anyone has ever said that to me. The doctors only told me that surgery would either work or it wouldn't – but nobody ever told me I was OK. That really makes me feel so relieved. You've helped me more in 5 minutes than my doctors have done in 6 months."

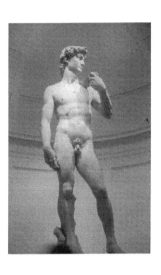

"Perfection" is a word derived from the ancient Latin *perfectio* meaning, "complete" or "lacking nothing." I am often asked if I really believe this is true, if I believe that we are all really perfect. Obviously, the *experience* of being inherently perfect is rare. Most of the time we walk around with the aches, diseases and dissatisfactions that feel like evidence that there really is something wrong with us. (This is why the Conventional approach seems so reasonable.) Yet I find little uplifting or empowering in going through life with an underlying belief that I am inherently broken or dysfunctional. So whether one really believes that they are perfect isn't really the point.

The point is the notion of "being perfect" is a starting place, an empowering *a priori* assumption. After all, the purpose of all the healthy life practices we adopt is to *increase* our sense of vitality and joyful personal power. Starting out with the assumption that we're perfect and whole creates the space for a whole new set of practices, vocabulary, methodologies, approaches and measurements, different than those found in the Conventional approach.

But to be entirely truthful, yes – I absolutely believe that we are all inherently perfect. It is our human nature to be complete and wanting nothing. We are born with the capacity for thought, emotion, movement and work, and connection to the Divine. We are by definition the marvelous interweaving of bodies, minds and Spirits. You can't be improved or fixed, because you can't get better than perfect! The purpose, therefore, of working out, eating well and managing stress is to take steps to *un*conceal our already-existing perfection.

These are the two halves of the Holistic approach in a nutshell. First, distinguish where your wholeness is concealed. Then reveal your perfection – literally "un-mask" it – in a way that has it live fully in your own experience, and in the experience of others.

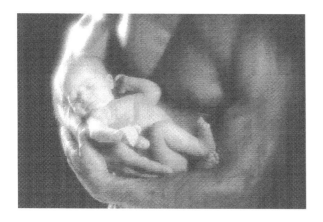

Physical Culture

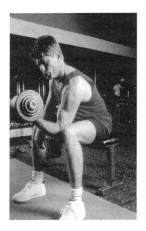

If you take a look, you'll find that part of the background of our modern world is a subtle conversation about our physical bodies. This conversation goes on inside our own heads, and tacitly between us and other people. Most importantly, this exchange takes place between us and our institutions of the body (like the media, our government agencies and our schools). The conversation goes something like this: being fit is attractive, and looks a certain way. Women are trim and busty; men are tall and muscular. Being fit is equated to being healthy, which is an intelligent thing to be. It takes time and discipline to be fit, an attribute of successful people. In other words, people who look fit are healthy, attractive, smart and successful. By contrast, people who don't look fit must be unhealthy, are unattractive, unintelligent and unsuccessful. This conversation is society's *weltenshauung* (world-view) of our bodies, something I call the prevailing "physical culture."

Comedian Billy Crystal once created a character named Fernando who told everyone they looked "mah-velous! And as you know," Fernando pointed out, "it is better to *look* good than to *feel* good." That's funny as a joke. But looking good (or performing better) is at the heart of our current physical culture – and that's no joke.

I want to make something clear at the outset of this book. I am not criticizing the current physical culture for the way it is. But it is enlightening to recognize that it is our physical culture that has given us the most available options for pursuing a healthy life. Where do you turn when you look for education or support in how to live longer, feel good about yourself, or be free of pain and disease? The institutions (like hospitals and universities), the training environments (like spas and fitness centers), the helpers (like doctors, nutritionists, therapists and personal trainers), the prescriptions and protocols, and even the very theories behind what it means to be fit and healthy arise from our current conversation of the body.

There is nothing wrong with this conversation. It's just that this conversation is so prevalent it is virtually the only conversation there is. The appearance of fitness can be deceiving; beauty that is only skin deep may hide a life out of balance. The Holistic approach is fundamentally about being *in* balance, and that may look very different on different people. So I want to make sure my message here is clear: *there is nothing wrong with looking trim and athletic.*

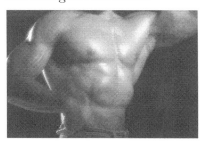

But if you look closely, you will discover that our current physical culture actually *excludes* a majority of our population, and chases them away from participating in health-related practices. For the purposes of this book, we'll call the practices that arise from our current physical culture the Conventional approach – the contrast to the Holistic approach. I wrote this book specifically because I believe the Conventional approach is a "glass half-empty" way of looking at life. I, on the other hand, am a disciple of the "glass half-full" way of looking at the world. For more than half my life, I have applied that perspective to the question of what it means to be fit, well and healthy. This book is my way of sharing the answers I've come up with. My goal – my wish, my invitation – is that you'll take the insights in this book and use them. Build on them and teach them to others. With these ideas as a starting place, make new discoveries I've not thought of, and lead us all into the future world of which I dream.

What's Going On?

In 1995 the US Surgeon General's office issued a landmark paper entitled, "A Report on Health and Physical Activity." According to this report, fewer than 20% of Americans get the minimum amount of daily physical activity to maintain good health. The report likened the lack of daily activity to smoking a pack of cigarettes a day. More than 250,000 people die every year from conditions arising directly from not getting enough exercise.

What was the impact of the Surgeon General's report? Since the release of the Surgeon General's report in 1995, diabetes, obesity and inactivity have actually *increased* in America. Heart disease, mental illness and cancer – the three leading causes of death in our country – are also on the rise.

Ask any doctor – or for that matter any grandmother – and she will tell you that the best medicine is *preventive* medicine. Preventive medicine is really nothing more than good sense living – eating well, resting enough, and getting plenty of physical exercise. It's the kind of good common sense that everyone knows and most people believe in.

Yet 80% of Americans still do not get even the *minimum* amount of daily physical activity to maintain good health. Obesity for both children and adults in America has reached epidemic proportion. Stress related death, including suicide, is now ranked as the #2 cause for early mortality among all Americans, and the leading cause of death among adolescents and teens. In short, most Americans are not taking care to live sensibly.

Why is it that most people in America today are inactive, or inattentive to their diet and stress management? Personally, I do *not* believe it's because they are lazy, or ignorant of the importance and impact of good health practices. After twenty-five years of work in the fitness industry, I believe that most Americans are inactive because our current fitness practices and environments exclude the average person, and drive them away from participating in physical activity, good nutrition and stress management.

For example, I've looked closely at why people avoid exercise. I have observed that it is most often for one or more of these four common reasons:

1) because they are not motivated by reaching goals, which is still the most common way exercise is presented;

2) because their bodies don't feel good doing the kinds of workouts our industry offers to them;

3) because their self-image does not match the models promoted by the fitness media and our physical culture; or

4) because they don't see the connection to the beautiful synergy of their body, mind and Spirit.

Of course, neither the Conventional approach nor the Holistic approach is inherently more *true* or *real* than the other. Each different approach simply operates on a specific set of *a priori* assumptions, and these assumptions each give rise to a distinct set of practices. However, I believe that the Holistic approach is more complete, and therefore likely to be more effective in making perfect health available to more people. For one thing, being more complete, the Holistic approach avoids the physical and emotional omissions that lead to chronic illness, pain and early death.

Two Differing Paradigms

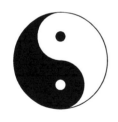

The Holistic approach to fitness, wellness and health differs from what is common in the Fitness industry in a number of ways. In order to understand the differences (and similarities) among workouts, diets and stress management techniques, we need to understand *why* these methods are designed the way they are. After all, these methods don't grow on trees; they are invented and taught by people. We might ask, then, how do the people who invent workouts etc. see the human body, and by what yardstick do they measure their effects on the human body? Well, consider that each approach (Holistic and Conventional) operates from its own particular paradigm – its matrix of organizing principles, images and references. The first step in understanding a new Holistic way of looking at your life and your health is to understand the current, Conventional paradigm.

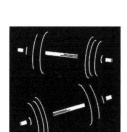

Understanding the salient features of the two approaches – Conventional and Holistic – will help you make more powerful choices. For example, do you look forward with excitement to the idea of eating well every day – including shopping and preparing your meals? Do workouts feel more like work or play? When you face the challenges of your day, do you feel closer to your Spirit, or do you feel like you've left a part of yourself at home?

The characteristics of the Conventional approach have set up the exercise, nutrition and stress management practices with which we are so familiar. Remember, the more we compartmentalize ourselves (by getting too specific, goal-oriented, stimulated or outwardly-directed) the farther away we move from balance. The farther from balance we move, the more we conceal our inherent perfection.

Why then would anyone ever operate out of the Conventional approach? Simply put, the Conventional approach is inherently competitive, stimulating and specific, and many people are temperamentally drawn to these characteristics. They will find bliss in these workouts. Still other people will benefit therapeutically from Conventional-style exercises, for example the ones that efficiently correct balance. But let's get a little more specific and look at the details of the two paradigms.

The Conventional Paradigm

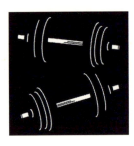

- ❖ The Conventional Approach is Specific and Reductionist.
- ❖ The Conventional Approach is Goal-Oriented.
- ❖ The Conventional Approach is Stimulating to the Nervous System.
- ❖ The Conventional Approach is Concerned with Appearance and Performance.

The Conventional approach is the standard of our physical culture. It is fitness-based, scientific and reductionistic – which means it reduces the human body into a collection of parts, all with a special function, operating together like a fantastic machine. It is essentially a scientific approach and parallels the Conventional Western approach to medicine, which is our scientific model of how the human body works. Even the research done on exercise, nutrition and stress management is most often done in scientific environments, using Western medical measurement standards and recorded in Western medical terminologies.

> *"In a nutshell, physical activity is something you do. Physical fitness is something you acquire – a characteristic or an attribute one can achieve by being physically active. And exercise is structured and tends to have fitness as a goal."* -- Michael Pratt, MD; CDC Division of Nutrition and Physical Activity

Let's just take a look at one of the components of health: physical activity, also known as exercise. Conventional exercise professionals are "fix-it" specialists. A trainer's job, according to the Conventional paradigm, is to design a workout routine that will help you reach your peak of fitness. They analyze your body, finding its strengths and weaknesses, they help you set goals and they monitor your progress as your muscles get bigger, or you run farther, or you lose weight. On the following pages, let's examine the prominent features of the Conventional approach to exercise – which by the way are also the prominent features of the Conventional approach to nutrition and stress management.

Feature #1 -- Specificity

For most Conventional trainers, a workout is considered to be less valuable if it doesn't maximize results. To put this in context, it may help to know that most of what trainers "do" is modeled after either physical therapy or sports conditioning, and in particular body building. A competitive athlete doesn't just want to go faster, he wants to be the *fastest*. He or she doesn't just want to be big; he or she wants to be the *biggest*. Athletic training has led professional fitness trainers to develop the rule of isolation, which is the practice of focusing a workout on just one movement or body part to maximize results in specific locations. Body builders, for example, may focus on just one part of one muscle in one muscle group in one area of the body.

Feature #2 -- Goal Orientation

The second most distinctive characteristic of the Conventional paradigm is goal-orientation. One of the first questions fitness professionals are taught to ask is, "What are your goals?" If you don't have any, or don't know how to articulate them, that's ok – we'll help you by giving you three choices. Would you like to lose weight, tone up, or build muscle?

To succeed in athletic competition is, by definition, to pursue and achieve a goal. The Conventional approach to exercise values results, and emphasizes the products of our labor, rather than the labor itself. Conventional workouts focus on the mechanics of exercise, as in, "What does this movement do for this part of your body?" The goal of Conventional exercise is the development of strength, flexibility, speed and power.

Jim, a retired Catholic priest I know, told me he stopped going to health clubs because they were too competitive. Even in family-oriented fitness centers, he pointed out, you can't get away from high powered music, the aggressive clanking of metal weights, and the sounds of men and women grunting and straining.

It's a subtle kind of competitiveness, hidden by the fact there is no finish line to cross, no points on a scoreboard. But just below the surface there is an attitude of, "How much weight is that guy lifting? I'll bet I can lift more!" or "I think my abs are a lot flatter than hers." In fact, fitness trainers teach their clients to be competitive – although you're supposed to learn to compete against your own performance.

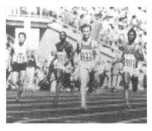

By the way, the Conventional approach to diet has the same kind of goal-orientation. A diet is really nothing more that a structured way to take in nutritious food to keep the body vital and vibrant. Most of the time, however, we think of a diet as a way to achieve a goal – losing or gaining weight.

Feature #3 -- Stimulation
Conventional workouts are characteristically emotionally exciting and physically stimulating. This is no accident. Fundamental to the Conventional approach is a theory of stress called the General Adaptation Syndrome (GAS). This principle says that if you challenge your body to do more work than it normally does, the body will adapt, change and grow to become able to handle the new work demand – or it will die. In other words, adding stress to the body is inherent to the Conventional approach.

First put forth by Dr. Hans Selye, the General Adaptation Syndrome theory states that when an organism encounters a stressor, it responds in three stages. The first stage is the "Alarm Stage." Here the organism first recognizes that something is going on, and begins to react to it. Some reactions of the Alarm stage – like the fear reaction – are almost instantaneous. These reactions and alarms are meant to protect the body from danger and imminent harm, and alert the other bodily systems to be ready to act.

The second stage is the "Resistance Stage." In this stage, the organism continues to react to the stressor, but now specifically it responds by changing and adapting itself to meet the challenge of the stressor. In other words, the organism, sensing that it is being attacked by something that could potentially cause it harm, starts to reshape itself (gets stronger, shorter, tighter, bigger) in order to "resist" or protect itself.

The third and final stage is the "Exhaustion Stage." Here the stressor is coming too fast, or in too large a volume, for the organism to change or resist fast enough. The organism tried to cope, but can't keep up. This is when injury usually happens.

Conventional training uses the GAS as its model, manipulating the intensity, frequency or duration of the stressor so that the body is forced to change, grow and strengthen. Trainers walk the fine line between just the right amount of a stressor to keep someone in the Resistance Stage, or too much of a stress to throw the organism into exhaustion.

There can be a down side to the high intensity workouts that are so common in Conventional exercise. These workouts and the environments in which they are done are also "anxiety causing," and characteristically result in activation of the sympathetic nervous system. This is your "fight or fight" response, accompanied by higher blood pressure, elevated heart rate, increased adrenaline levels in the blood and higher levels of norepinephrine and dopamine (the neurotransmitters of stress and aggression) in the brain.

Feature #4 -- Appearance

Finally, the Conventional exercise paradigm is typically outer-directed, as in "how do I appear to others?" Many people take up exercise to lose weight not because they want to be healthier, but because it will make them look more attractive. But like clothing fashions that change from season to season, Conventional workouts tend to be "faddish," changing from year to year to keep people interested, motivated and entertained.

The Holistic Paradigm

- ❖ The Holistic Approach is focused on Synergy.
- ❖ The Holistic Approach is Process-orientated.
- ❖ The Holistic Approach is Energy-centric.
- ❖ The Holistic Approach elicits The Relaxation Response.

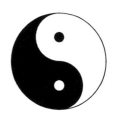

Obviously, not everyone is drawn to the Conventional approach. If they were, most people would be working out regularly, eating well, and thriving on stress and I wouldn't be writing this book. The truth is, few people in America are motivated by the Conventional paradigm. Here is a grand oversimplification: with respect to motivation, there are basically two types of people in the world. There are those who are goal-oriented, and those who are process-oriented.

Most of the professionals in the exercise and weight loss industries are accustomed to serving people who are motivated by results. These customers are relatively easy to attract and keep in our typical exercise environments. These people are physical by nature and like to be active. They are also characteristically at ease with the mechanics of Conventional workout routines. They are attracted to the idea of relieving stress through physical activity.

The Holistic approach, on the other hand, transforms working out into a process of discovering both self and health. Increasingly, Americans are drawn to seek ways to become more synergistic, more whole. They are drawn to wellness and health, not to fitness.

As we saw in the Surgeon General's report, the Conventional approach is working for less than a third of the adults in the United States. Far more representative of the majority of people in America are those who are motivated by process more than by results. For these people, stress is better relieved through *feeling* rather than doing. Workouts, selected on the basis of an individual's BodyMind type (more on this presently), can and should incorporate the mind and Spirit just as much as they work the body. They respond better to exercise that feels "soulful" rather than mechanical. Here are the prominent features of the Holistic approach to exercise, which are also the prominent features of the Holistic approach to nutrition and stress management.

In the Holistic approach, authenticity lies not in the end product, but in the *process*. The purpose of a workout is not necessarily to achieve a specific goal or result, although there are important and measurable effects of every movement. The purpose, if that is an appropriate word, is simply *to do it*. The reward is in the journey itself, not in the destination. Also, the Holistic paradigm creates workouts specifically designed to get the parts of the body to work together and to synergize the body's motions with the thoughts and images held in the mind. Holistic workouts focus less on the "mechanical" aspects of exercise like strength, speed or flexibility, and more on the concept of the "energy" which underlies the ability to do the movement. Holistic workouts tend to be cooperative rather than competitive in nature, and sedating rather than stimulating, often activating the parasympathetic nervous system.

Feature #1 -- Synergy

While the Conventional paradigm is characterized by its focus on isolation, specificity and results, the Holistic paradigm focuses on synergy and inner experience. In other words, in contrast to the Conventional exercise paradigm, within the Holistic paradigm we find workouts specifically designed to get the parts of the body to work together, and to join together the body's motions with the thoughts and images held in the mind.

I was introduced to the mind/body approach in an unusually profound way. In the late 1970's, I had decided to take a T'ai Chi class just to see what it was like. I knew almost nothing about T'ai Chi Ch'uan, and I had never been very **athletic** before then. I was not prepared for what was about to happen. On the first day of class, as I was stumbling along, trying to follow the movements of my teacher, I was suddenly overcome by a rush of heat that spread throughout my body in a flash. I felt as though every cell in my body was a living, breathing entity and I was in touch with them all. And more than that, I felt connected with the whole world around me. For the space of those few moments, I saw colors more vibrantly than I can ever remember seeing them before or since.

I know now that I was experiencing an intense sudden circulation of the inner life energy, called *ch'i* in Chinese medicine. The experience lasted only moments, but it changed my life completely. The feeling of complete integration was so profound, it gave me a yardstick by which to measure my personal health and a new perspective on exercise. Working out, I realized for the first time, can make you feel *alive!*

Holistic exercise includes all of the mechanical components found in Conventional workouts. It develops strength, like weight lifting; it improves the cardiovascular system, like running; it expands flexibility, like gymnastics. But Holistic exercise goes further than Conventional exercise by involving the mind and the Spirit. Ruth Stricker, who owns The Marsh, a pioneering mind/body center in Minneapolis, says Holistic exercise helps to develop, "simultaneous awareness of the body and the psychological self, coupled with a simultaneous enhanced awareness of what is happening around you."

While the Conventional paradigm is characterized by its focus on isolation, specificity and results, the Holistic paradigm focuses on integration and inner experience. In other words, in contrast to the Conventional exercise paradigm, within the Holistic paradigm we find workouts specifically designed to get the parts of the body to work together, and to "integrate" the body's motions with the thoughts and images held in the mind.

Feature #2 -- Process-Orientation

In the Holistic paradigm, wholeness and balance resides not in the end product, but in the process. The Holistic approach to exercise is a process-oriented approach. The purpose of a workout is not necessarily to achieve a specific goal or result, although there are important and measurable effects of every movement. The *purpose*, if that is an appropriate word, is simply to do it. The reward is in the journey itself, not in the destination.

Feature #3 -- Energy-Centric

Holistic workouts also focus less on the *"mechanical"* aspects of exercise like strength, speed or flexibility, and more on the concept of the *"energy"* which underlies the ability to do movement. This energy, called by many names like ch'i, ki, or prana, is what activates the changes in the body. But unlike the Conventional paradigm, which sees change as a process of adaptation, the Holistic paradigm sees change as a process of revelation.

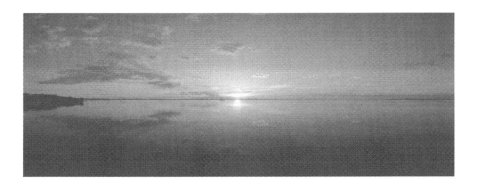

Feature #4 -- The Relaxation Response

When we first looked at the features of the Conventional approach, we noticed that one of fundamental concepts is the General Adaptation Syndrome, which says that if you apply stress to an organism it will either adapt or die. Many fitness professionals have used this concept as though it meant the more stress you add to the body, the more results you will get. Yet this is not necessarily the case. There is another fundamental principle, known as the "Yerkes-Dodson Law of Arousal." According to this principle, stress – or "arousal" as it is called here – improves performance up to a certain point. After that point, performance actually declines with continued stress. In other words, muscles could get weaker, organs could get injured, and anxiety could worsen.

Holistic workouts tend to be calming rather than stimulating, often activating the parasympathetic nervous system. These workouts are based on *reducing* and *relieving* the stress to the body, which is inherent in the principle of relaxation. One result is to reverse the downhill curve on the Yerkes-Dodson bell graph, improving performance and generating greater results.

Conventional	*Holistic*
Dissociative	Synergistic
Beta brainwaves	Alpha brainwaves
Result Oriented	Process Oriented
Competitive	Cooperative
Doing	Feeling
Sympathetic NS	Parasympathetic NS
Depletes immunity	Increases immunity
Outer directed	Inner directed
Left brain	Right brain

Power, Freedom and Flow

So what, you might ask, does the Holistic approach actually give me? Beyond the theory of being complete and perfect, what tangible benefits does it have? Specifically, the Holistic approach is meant to alter your experience of life. Later in this book, you will learn about specific practices that lead you to balance, and spark moments of *feeling* complete and perfect. As you begin to feel balanced, perfect and complete, you will experience yourself and your life in a particular way – namely you will experience the presence of **Power, Freedom and Flow**.

Power is *vitality* – literally, the experience of the vital life energy flowing through your body, mind and Spirit. Power is the ability to cause an outcome without the use of strength or force. This is an important distinction: power is not the same thing as strength or force. For example, power flows, but force does not. Power is inclusive, releasing, and unlimited; strength and force carry the sense of holding onto or resisting something and have their limits.

By the same token, **Freedom** is boundless, uninhibited *acceptance*. Freedom is not constrained in any way, neither by memories of the past, nor by circumstances of the present, nor even by projections of the future.

Finally, **Flow** is the sense of uninterrupted *continuity* and *connectedness*. It is what athletes call the "sweet spot," or "being in the zone." Flow often brings with it a sense of timelessness, effortless action and the "runners' high." Flow is not self-conscious, nor is it passive, awkward or aggressive.

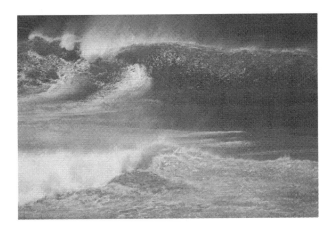

Masks of the BodyMind

So why is it that we are not all walking around in a state of integrity, compassion and synergy all the time? If we're all perfect and complete, why don't we experience power, freedom and flow?

A baby is born into this world a perfect miracle of life. At birth, he or she hasn't yet experienced rejection, failure, disappointment or shame. A baby lives moment to moment without any self-imposed constraints on its self-expression. From age two until just before adolescence (and the onset of teenage gawkiness), a child is an unstoppable bundle of motion and synergy, able to climb trees, swing off a rope into a river, or mimic the most complex dances without effort. From the time they awaken until they reluctantly succumb to sleep, a child experiences the power of life's energy without even thinking of it, the way a fish swims in water without knowing it is wet.

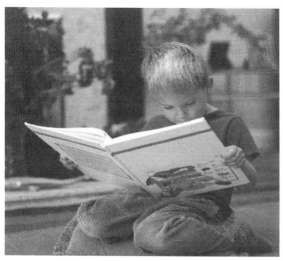

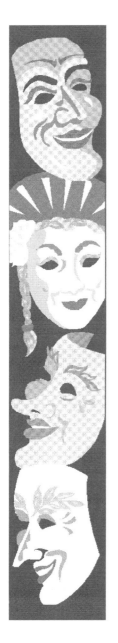

Somewhere along the path of growing up, however, life begins to occur as a series of disappointments, compromises and dangers. We lose the sense of power, freedom and flow we had as children. Yet despite our feelings of frustration, isolation or struggle the only thing we ever really lose is a certain *experience*. We never fall from grace, or somehow become less than perfect. We merely cover over our true nature with a series of masks.

A mask is essentially a compensation we create for ourselves to make up for a place where we lost the experience of being connected from body to mind to Spirit. We create this compensation because in some way we think it will afford us greater functionality, or more Power, Freedom and Flow. The thing is, these compensations are actually the *breakdown* of functionality and a wall between us and the experience of Power, Freedom and Flow. Every mask we create widens the gap between the *actuality* of our inner perfection and our moment-to-moment *experience* of it. Soon the gap is so wide that all we show others is the mask, and all that we see in the mirror is our disguise.

Revelation

The Holistic approach starts with the process of exploration; we have to "discover" the whole person that we are. In searching for our complete, authentic selves, we'll recognize not only that much of the time the whole person is concealed, hidden or masked, but we also begin to see *why* it is concealed. Health, happiness and self-actualization are all inherent within us. They are the faces of the soul. The Holistic philosophy is that one doesn't "create" health or happiness; one learns to "disappear" the barriers that prevent their natural and effortless occurrence.

Discovery, therefore, is the process of revelation, distinguishing what might be concealing your perfection. What conceals our perfection can be seen as the degree to which we have stepped away from balance, or the degree to which we've reduced ourselves into parts. Later in this book you're going to learn to use some simple techniques to reveal what's hidden behind what we think we see about ourselves. You will explore the most common and fundamental types of masks we typically construct, how to recognize them by the symptoms they cause on the physical level, and how to understand those symptoms not only literally but also metaphorically.

When you look at yourself in the mirror, you see a unique physical tapestry, woven by the history of your life's events. Your personal tapestry may portray a body of muscular imbalances and weaknesses, varying degrees of flexibility and balance, a lifted shoulder here, an off-kilter hip over there, and toes that turn out severely down on the ground. In Chapter IV, you will actually learn how to interpret what you see in the mirror in a way that will allow you to build a program for dissolving the masks that conceal your wholeness.

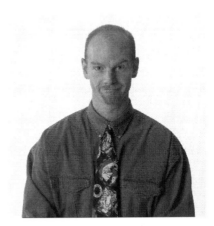

Exercise

I am often struck by how difficult it is even for holistic wellness professionals to break out of the Conventional paradigm. At a recent seminar, one of my students asked, "Once we've identified our clients' masks and compensations, how do we fix them?"

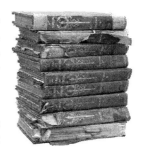

I stopped her right there, and reminded her that the Holistic approach was not about "fixing" anything, but rather "uncovering" what was hidden.

"Got it," she said. "What I meant to say was, how do we go about suggesting the appropriate *corrections*?" She realized what she had said as soon as the words left her mouth. She laughed, smacked herself on the forehead with the heel of her palm and said, "You know what I mean!"

The difficulty comes from the fact that we don't have a working vocabulary for a healing paradigm in which nothing is seen as "wrong." How can we expect the Holistic paradigm to be distinguished as unique, workable and relevant when we continue to use the language of the Conventional paradigm? Below is a list of words frequently used in the context of the Conventional approach. In the space provided across from those words, write your own Holistic alternatives. For example, instead of fitness, I talk about wellness.

Conventional Language	Holistic Alternatives
Fitness	Wellness
Trainer	
Cardio	
Cure	
Treatment	
Workout	
Correction	
Gym	
Diet	

A Final Thought

At a recent seminar for yoga teachers, I was working with a student on a pose called *Uttanasana* -- the standing forward bend. She was folded over at the hips, with her head down by her knees, and I was gently pushing her forward so that her body weight would be over the middle of her feet, rather than on her heels. "Stop!" she said. "I'm going to fall over!" The thing is, she wasn't anywhere close to falling over forward – in fact she was leaning slightly backward. However, her *proprioceptors* (those sensory nerves which help us orient in space and motion) were sending signals that her rational mind interpreted as tipping forward. Interpretation is an invention the mind makes up to explain things, and sometimes the story is very different from what's really there. In other words, her mind was masking the posture that was truly there, hiding it from her view.

In a way, most of us are like my yoga student, looking at the world upside down, and operating from the Conventional assumption that we are always about to fall over – that there is something wrong with us that needs to be fixed or improved. There is nothing wrong with looking at the world upside down. Moreover, if you look around and everyone else seems to be hanging onto the same belief, then that seems like the most reasonable point of view.

But we could just as easily say that authentic, holistic living starts with the supposition that we are all perfect, whole and complete. Anything that doesn't look or feel perfect is just perfection concealed. In other words, perfection isn't missing – it is there – it's just sometimes hidden from view. Your rational mind is misinterpreting the information that your senses and emotions are sending you. And buying into the perception that something is wrong diminishes the soul – your connection with your authentic inner self.

What kind of view does the Holistic approach give you? Essentially, the Holistic approach is meant to expose you to an experience of life that goes beyond the merely physical. The Conventional approach has given us a scientific education about the health benefits of wellness, but that is information for your head. To actually have the *experience* of power, freedom and flow in your body is to feel healthy on every level of your being. Holistic living, therefore, is *soulful* living – where soul is the word I give to the conscious moment-by-moment awareness of being perfect and complete, and life feels like the miraculous interweaving of body, thoughts, emotions and Spirit.

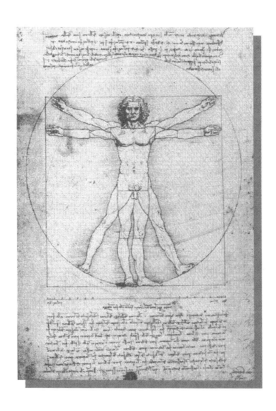

Chapter II: The Five Seasons of the BodyMind

The gift of the second chapter, The 5 Seasons, is *acceptance*. In this chapter you will distinguish the unique characteristics that make you who you are. Open this gift, and I hope to hear you say, "Because I now understand *myself* better, I finally see that people really are different – and it's okay for me to be me!"

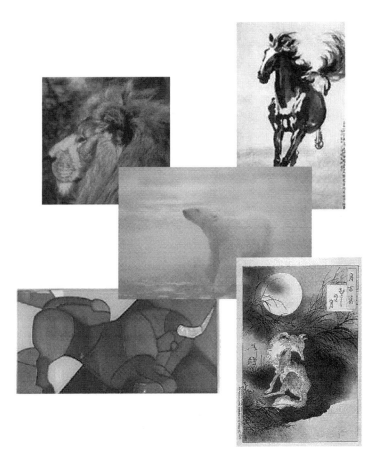

`Who are YOU?' said the Caterpillar.

This was not an encouraging opening for a conversation. Alice replied, rather shyly, `I--I hardly know, sir, just at present-- at least I know who I WAS when I got up this morning, but I think I must have been changed several times since then.'

`What do you mean by that?'* said the Caterpillar sternly. *`Explain yourself!'

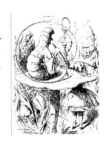

Who Are You?

Many years ago, when I was in college, my friends and I used to play a game called, "What's their major?" It's a people-watching game, and it went like this: my friends and I would wait until someone interesting walked by, and as they passed we'd turn to each other and ask, "What's their major?"

For example, if a slim, demure looking girl with glasses and an armload of books walked by, we'd say, "English Lit." On the other hand, if it was a somewhat overweight guy with a bad haircut, wearing a plaid shirt and polyester pants, we'd say, "Computer Science." The easiest ones of all were the guys wearing jeans and polo shirts, new Nike shoes and carrying only a slim notebook. "Phys. Ed!" we'd cry.

Of course, we were practicing the most blatant form of stereotyping. We didn't have any idea whether the people we pegged as International Finance majors weren't really Drama students.

On the other hand, there was *something* we felt we recognized about the way they carried themselves, the way they dressed, the expressions in their eyes, whether they walked alone or in pairs or in groups, which made us think they were a certain "type" of person.

Diversity means different people deserve different approaches and methods. Consider that human beings experience their world simultaneously on all human levels – physically, emotionally, intellectually and spiritually. Moreover, two people may experience the same event in profoundly different ways. Part of that experience is given by conditioning (their past and likely future), in other words the way they have *learned* to process information. But another part of that experience is given by the senses and temperaments they were born with -- the way they are *genetically predisposed* to process information.

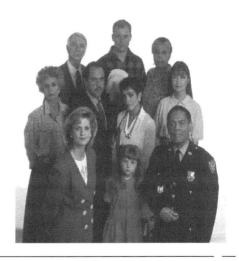

Understanding diversity is a fundamental part of the Holistic approach. By being able to understand our individual and unique needs, drives and desires, we can better predict the likelihood of success, failure or comfort level. Since many of us come to the practices of fitness, wellness or health for the first time – or return to them after a long absence – doesn't it make sense to create a powerful and inspiring first experience?

First impressions are lasting impressions, and first experiences are critical experiences. The more accurately we can predict what our responses to a new diet or activity are likely to be, then we can steer ourselves toward experiences that are likely to be more comfortable or successful. And with initial success comes the likelihood that we will stick to our new diet or workout until it becomes a deeply ingrained lifestyle habit.

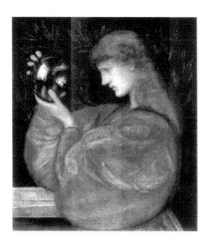

Recognizing Mind/Body Types

In fact, you could probably think of a number of stereotypes that fit certain people you know -- the introverted, serious, sedentary accountant; or the plump, smiling, always loving grandmother. Your own experience will probably tell you that people share certain characteristics with others that make them more alike than they are different, and these characteristics are so distinct anybody can recognize them. In other words, people seem to posses a recognizable set of physical and personality characteristics. An individual's unique combination of mental and physical characteristics makes for an identifiable "psycho-physiological profile" – or "BodyMind type."

Let's look at this principle another way. The first step in designing a truly Holistic program for fitness, wellness or health is to determine what makes you unique. One way to do that is to distinguish in what way you are similar to others who share your traits and characteristics. As you explore Holistic options, you will discover that some alternatives easily click for you and others just don't, and you may wonder, "why?" Many people have asked me over the years, "What's the *best* workout (or diet, or stress management technique)?" My answer is typically: "The one you'll do again tomorrow."

Even the most comprehensive and efficient exercise regimen will not be effective if no one does it. Imagine that you had access to a system that would aid you in predicting what your responses were likely to be, given a certain set of stimuli. Now you could actually make more powerful choices in the techniques you select, steering yourself towards experiences that are likely to be more comfortable and successful. The goal: to make the lifestyle practices of fitness, wellness and health irresistibly fun and effective.

Personality and Temperament

Each of us actually has two sets of mind/body characteristics. First of all, each of us has an intrinsic nature with which we are born, as fundamental as our eye color or fingerprints. But we can also acquire certain traits as we grow, traits we learn depending on our jobs, families or school environments. Dr. Dean Hamer, a researcher at the National Cancer Institute and author of the book *Living With Our Genes*, calls it the difference between "temperament" and "character."

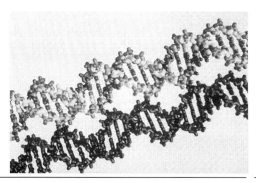

Temperament, says Hamer, is deep and intrinsic. It's what we're born with, what we get from our parents. In other words, our temperament is genetic. On the other hand, character is a more surface expression of who we are. What Hamer calls character, I prefer to call "personality."

In many people, the personality is roughly the same as the temperament. But others will have developed personality characteristics more common to a different temperament. Often people will do this to survive in a stressful environment, or to achieve success in a job dominated by a certain temperament different from their own. But down deep, there is always an unchanging inner core. It is this inner core that is the true BodyMind type.

The theory of BodyMind types tells us it is possible to predict someone's personality -- the way that people process information, make decisions and become internally motivated -- by observing their body, and taking note of certain physical, somatic-based information. In the same way, by observing someone's emotional and intellectual characteristics, it is possible to predict the ways their body will react to stress, foods and physical activity.

Generic workouts, like generic diets or generic medicine, don't work for everyone. So what is it that keeps people exercising? According to Dr. Jay Kimiciek, if you ask people who are "regular exercisers" why they continue to work out consistently, they are most likely to answer, "because I like it," or "because I feel good." They rarely, if ever, say they do it because they know it will make them more fit. These people have made the move, says Dr. Kimiciek, from being extrinsically motivated (exercising because they think somehow they should) to being intrinsically motivated (exercising because they are emotionally inspired to do it from deep within). The move from extrinsic to intrinsic motivation is they key factor in becoming a regular exerciser.

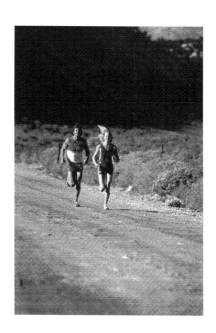

But what may be an intrinsic motivator for one person may not be at all inspiring for another person. In other words, what may feel soulful and integrative to me may be boring, exasperating or even stressful to you. Each of us has an identifiable set of physical, mental and emotional characteristics – a 'psycho-physiological profile." To know a person's profile is to know something important about them, like how their bodies react to working out, to eating various foods, and to experiencing emotional stress. It also tells me what a person's inner motivations are likely to be, how they gather information, and how they relate to other people. These are precisely the things I need to know about someone if I am to design a workout that gets them into exercise and keeps them there.

Fortunately, although everyone is unique and different, we are enough alike that we can be loosely separated in similar groups. In other words, there aren't six billion totally and completely different psycho-physiological profiles -- there are only five. We call them the Five-Season BodyMind types. The temperamental traits that are shared by members of each mind/body type make each type more likely to enjoy (subjectively) and benefit (objectively) from certain types of exercise as opposed to other types of exercise. Knowing your type is one of the best ways to make an intelligent choice about exercise. This is really the starting point for selecting a workout that will inspire and fulfill you.

The History of Typing

"Typing" -- the practice of understanding people according to their shared temperamental and personality characteristics -- has been around a long time. Throughout history, various cultures have evolved unique systems for recognizing and naming them. In ancient India, the medical tradition of Ayurveda recognized the combination of three "doshas." In China, their traditional healing art was based on the theory that people are influenced (and therefore can be typed) by the five basic elements of the universe -- wood, fire, water, earth and metal.

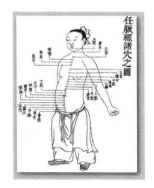

Both Ayurveda and traditional Chinese medicine devised their typologies by combining generations of observation with their ancient theories about the nature of the basic elements and energies of the universe. As each respective system evolved, the characteristics that describe people became more distinct and defined, until they could definitely describe distinct archetypes. But these two systems can and do use an interactive survey to determine type (like the questionnaire you'll find in the appendix). However, the more accurate method used by clinicians is *pulse diagnosis*.

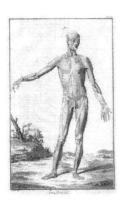

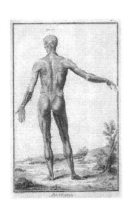

Whereas questionnaires are subjective, pulse diagnosis is objective. In fact, it works consistently enough to have accurately predicted states of illness and to have determined appropriate treatments for thousands of years.

Another objective system is "somatyping." When I was in school, I learned to look at human bodies as ectomorphic, mesomorphic or endomorphic. The advantage of this kind of typing is that you know it will be consistent. An endomorph today will be an endomorph in a decade, and will be an endomorph in Tokyo or London. On the other hand, this method of typing says absolutely nothing about psychological characteristics. In terms of describing a total mind and body combination, it is incomplete.

Hippocrates, the Greek physician who is honored as the "Father of Western Medicine," proclaimed that people were one of four types, the Sanguine, the Choleric, the Melancholy and the Phlegmatic. The "Personality Plus" system was originally based on the four personalities described by Hippocrates and, like Ayurveda and Chinese medicine, were originally based on observation. This system appeals to many. "Yes, I know a sanguine," you say. But these four types seemed simplistic to me, and I wondered if this system was only describing varying degrees of introversion and extroversion.

Perhaps the most well known system of typing used by modern Western psychologists and social workers is the Myers-Briggs Type Indicator (MBTI), a system based on the work of Carl Jung. The MBTI groups people based on the combination of four pairs of complementary attributes: introversion v. extroversion; sensing v. intuition; thinking v. feeling; and judging v. perceiving.

The MBTI was originally based on Jung's observation that human personality could be described by the degree of introversion, information gathering styles, decision-making habits, and degree of objectivity v. subjectivity. But then the system seems to become a math game or an exercise in logic. The four pairs of characteristics becomes a table of 16 possible combinations.

The team of Sandra Seagal and David Horne developed one of the most impressive new systems I've seen. It is called "Human Dynamics," and it is based on the theory that human personality comprises the three aspects of the physical, mental and emotional. They way that these aspects combine in an individual defines their particular "dynamic." For example, if a person primarily gathers information in a "mental" way, and the information they are most interested in gathering is about the "physical," objectified world, they are called a "mental-physical" dynamic.

According to Seagal and Horne, there is a possibility of nine different personality dynamics. But after 20 years of observation, and more than 40,000 interviews with people from 25 different countries worldwide, it seems that only five of these dynamics appear with enough regularity to be statistically important. This is concurrent with both ayurveda and Chinese medicine. In ayurveda, for example, there are nine possible combinations of the doshas (not counting a possible tenth, in which all three doshas are perfectly and equally present). In Chinese medicine, there are five elements, and physicians often refer to a patient as a "wood" type, or a "fire" type, for example.

Like Seagal and Horne, I've also observed five predominant dynamics -- or, as I call them, "BodyMind types." Of course, there are always exceptions, variation and uniqueness that you find in every individual. But at the same time, the five types are distinct enough to describe what I see in most people.

The 5 Seasons of the BodyMind

The 5-Season BodyMind Typology was developed to describe the most common ways in which human beings express their diversity. The typology was designed through a meta-analysis of dozens of different typologies, including Ayurvedic typing, Chinese 5 Element theory, Meyers-Briggs, and Human Dynamics, just to name a few.

The 5 Season system outlines 5 basic profiles, or archetypes (Spring, Summer, Indian Summer, Autumn and Winter), and the Five Season typology describe some very practical attributes. Bear in mind that these attributes are genetically based, and therefore are more than the way people look or act because of conditioning.

The 5-Season typology tell us that it is possible to gain insight into your own personality – the way that you process information, make decisions, and become internally motivated – by observing you body, and taking note of certain physical, somatic-based information. In the same way, by observing someone's mental characteristics, it is possible to predict the ways your *body* will react to stress, foods or physical activity. Discovering your "Season" is the first step in the process of creating an effective program for yourself.

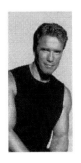

- Psycho-physio profile: The Warrior Spirit; typical Fitness Club Member/trainer; large mesomorph, strong musculature; good competitive athletes
- Intrinsic Motivator: Achievement/Action
- Inner Destabilizer: Ignores body's warning signs
- Reaction: Over-training
- Compatible Workouts: All workouts, particularly Conventional, fitness-based exercise. Benefits from goal setting process.

Spring - The Lion

Spring types are the quintessential go-getters, and their number one characteristic and intrinsic motivator is their initiative and drive for achievement. Springs are mavericks, pioneers, adventurers and entrepreneurs, but because they are also "take charge" kinds of people, they can often by found as leaders in business, medicine and politics. Spring types have a strong mental component to their temperament, and like to think that they have logical reasons for everything they do—although their decisions are just as likely to be based on emotion and "gut instinct." They are competitive and impatient, and others can sometimes interpret this as being pushy or controlling. Spring types, by the way, are typically the least likely to be interested in knowing about bodymind types.

Spring types love to brainstorm, and sometimes discussion with Spring types can be stormy indeed as thoughts fly back and forth, each questioning and expanding on each others' thoughts. Often this process results in unexpected revelations and new directions not considered before. On the other hand, Spring types have to be careful not to rush forward "half-cocked." Spring types benefit from learning how to set and achieve goals. The goal setting process, accompanied by step-by-step plans for achieving those goals, helps to bring the lofty visions of a Spring type down to earth. Goal setting provides a way to measure whether the actions of a Spring match their intentions.

Physically, Spring types tend to be medium boned and mesomorphic, though with a strong musculature. More squarely built than Summer types (who also tend to be mesomorphs), they make great competitive athletes, particularly in sports that require strength. However, Spring types need to be careful, because they can push themselves beyond their limits, ignoring the body's warning signs of impending injury or over-training. Once I was describing the Spring archetype to a client when he started nodding his head. "OK," I said, "I can tell you've got a story – what is it?"

"I was a tri-athlete," he said. "One day I was out running when I pulled my Achilles tendon. So I went to my doctor, who told me I needed to stay off it for at least six weeks. Well, after about two weeks I just couldn't stand it any more, and I went out for a run – and snapped my Achilles entirely. Now I'll never run another triathlon again."

Spring types love Conventional workouts, which satisfy their need for stimulation and a sense of achievement. Conventional workouts also produce measurable effects that satisfy Spring's goal-oriented attitudes. Most of the high-energy people in the Fitness Industry are Spring types. The best intrinsic motivator to get Spring types to become regular exercisers is the subtle sense of competition – even if it is against themselves.

Workouts like this are very motivating to the Spring types. At the same time, Spring types tend to lose focus, or to be distracted by the next challenge that comes along. The heat of competition is what sends Spring types out of balance. A good balancing strategy for Springs, therefore, is the practice of setting goals. Conventional personal trainers – who are themselves typically Spring types – recognize this about themselves, and find great success in their own lives when they use the goal setting process. This is why the Fitness industry has focused on goals so strongly – because it works so well for them!

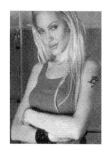

- ➢ Psycho-physio profile: The Free Spirit; small-medium mesomorph. Lean dancer's body; will try new, fun things.
- ➢ Intrinsic Motivator: Spontaneity
- ➢ Inner Destabilizer: Giving too much
- ➢ Reaction: Emotional burnout/mood swings
- ➢ Compatible Workouts: Hatha yoga, low-impact aerobics, dance, jazzercise, Nia, circuit-training

Summer - The Horse

The **Summer** type is characterized by their emotional spontaneity. The main organ of the Summer type - when we look at this type from the Chinese medicine point of view - is the heart, the organ of emotional thought Summer types are fiery, charismatic, dramatic; but also they are intensely loving and empathetic people. They often have a strong intuitive ability. They feel emotions strongly, both their own and those of others. They are great communicators, the life of the party, and often approach problem solving through "talking things out" At the same time, some people can view them as "touchy-feely."

Summer types are usually medium-boned and mesomorphic. They can make good athletes, dancers and gymnasts. Their skin, characteristically soft and moist, easily blushes. Summer types characteristically have an aversion to heat and are subject to digestive problems. They can also suffer from insomnia. In hot weather or in times of stress, they can overheat easily, and characteristically have a rapid pulse. Summer types have to watch out for circulatory problems.

Summer types tend to think of problems in terms of the people involved and how they are "feeling." They tend to personalize problems, but at the same time they are well able to handle concrete thinking and complex issues. For this reason, they dislike being patronized or being judged too emotional.

Summer types love to have fun, to do activities that involve other people. These activities don't necessarily have to have a particular goal in mind or end result - it is the *process* that inspires the Summer type more than the goal. In fact, here is a good contrast between Springs and Summers -- Springs get motivated and Summers get inspired. If a Summer type finds an aerobics teacher or a class with people they like, they often do well and become regular participants. But here again, it is because of the people involved, and not the activity itself. Certain workouts, however, seem to have the ability to draw out the strong emotional feelings on which Summer types thrive. Two good examples are NIA and Jazzercize.

Yvonne was a woman I met while I was director at Spa Ojai. A friend had given her a total spa package as a gift, and a personal training session with me was part of the package. Her resistance was evident on her face and in her body language when she walked into my office. She expected bad news, and she had already made up her mind that she wasn't going to like whatever I was going to tell her.

"I know I should be working out," she said with a sigh. "Every day I get into my car after work and tell myself I'm on my way to the gym. But I never get there." She paused and looked up at me. "You're probably going to make me lift weights, aren't you? How about if you just show me all the exercises really quick and then write it down for me so I can take it home."

"Actually," I said, "I was thinking of something entirely different. Let's start out by finding out what your BodyMind type is."

Yvonne turned out to be a Summer – charismatic, emotional and intuitive, with a medium to small bone structure, and a dancer's body. In fact, Yvonne told me that she had been a professional jazz and modern dancer when she was younger. As we read the Summer archetype together, I could see Yvonne's body language change. Her shoulders loosened, and she leaned in closer. I told her that Summer types, because of their extraverted nature, love to do things in groups. At the same time, however, because they are so loving, giving and emotional, their energy is always "going out." The most inspiring workouts for Summers, therefore, are workouts with a high fun factor, done with other people. The most balancing kinds of workouts for Summers are workouts with a calming, inner directed type of design, like yoga, group T'ai Chi, hiking, swimming or golf.

Now Yvonne was excited. "That's it exactly!" she exclaimed. "I've never like aerobics or weights – they always made me crazy. But I love yoga – I just never thought of it as a workout. Can you teach me a routine I can do on my own every day?"

The next day I saw Yvonne again. The yoga workout we had done together so inspired her that she had come back to the spa to work out a second time – on the weight machines. Then she had come back a third time to take a Pilates conditioning class. This was the woman who had dragged herself into my office, dreading the idea of exercise.

"I just want to tell you," she said, "I'm so sore from yesterday. But it kind of feels good, and I got up early this morning to practice my yoga routine – just so I don't forget!"

At the same time, Summer types are always outgoing, and it in fact the pouring out their own inner energy which sends Summer types out of balance. Balancing workouts for Summers, therefore, are ones which have an inner-directed or meditative component. Summer types need an opportunity to conserve their own inner energy and find inner peace. Group classes in hatha yoga and T'ai Chi Ch'uan often satisfy the dual needs for connection with people and meditation. Also, solo activities like walking and hiking, which gives Summer the chance to commune with Nature, and hear the echo of their own soul in the poetry of motion in a soulful environment.

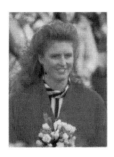

- Psycho-physio profile: The Nurturing Spirit; systemic thinkers; endomorph, slower metabolism, need to be early risers
- Intrinsic Motivator: Relationship
- Inner Destabilizer: Lethargy
- Reaction: Couch potato
- Compatible Workouts: Walking, jazzercise, T'ai Chi Ch'uan, swimming, tennis, cycling, circuit training

Indian Summer - The Bear

The **Indian Summer** type is known by their "down-to-earth" nature. Their most distinctive characteristic is how they find their identity in the group, whether it is family, church, occupation or politics. They tend to be larger boned and endomorphic -- real teddy bears -- and may tend toward a slower metabolism. Their skin is characteristically moist and clear, and their eyes large, bright and the whites liquid and clear. Early mornings make the best times for Indian Summer to exercise. In fact, this is a critical time for the Indian Summer type. If they get up and get active upon first awakening, they will do well and feel energetic for the rest of the day. On the other hand, if they lay in bed or fall back asleep, they may have trouble fully waking up, and may feel sluggish for the rest of the day.

The Indian Summer type may seem slow to get moving, but once they get started... watch out! They know exactly where they are going and are not likely to swerve from their path. They are "systemic thinkers," which means they see things from a Holistic point of view. They take their time gathering information, and once they see the whole picture, then they act decisively. Indian Summers are patient listeners, and extremely empathetic. They are the "family peacemakers," and often have trouble saying, "no."

Wendy, a very attractive 26-year old woman, wants to lose some weight. She looks good in her clothes, and she dresses fashionably, although she says she'd rather be a size 8 than a size 14. A few years ago, while living with a group of girls in a rented house for a summer, she slimmed down to her trimmest shape ever. She still keeps the jeans she bought that summer – a summer she spent eating fresh vegetable from the local farmers' market and riding her bicycle everywhere she went.

Since then, however, she's gained that weight back and actually gone up a few sizes. But Wendy has always been a "big girl," even as a child. Losing weight has always been a challenge for her. Yet in almost every other way, most people would call her a very healthy woman. She rarely gets sick, and she loves to dance and hike in the mountains. She tries to eat well, and she's been a vegetarian all her life.

The thing is, Wendy hates to "exercise." It's not that she's lazy or lethargic; she likes being active and out-of-doors. It is just the idea of going into a gym and lifting weights or walking on a treadmill that turns her off. But everything she's heard has led her to believe that the only way to slim down is to work out. So every January she goes down to join the local health club. And by Valentine's Day, she's stopped going.

Wendy is an Indian Summer. Although she has a sincere desire to lose weight, she's not truly motivated by reaching a certain goal. She's more motivated by people connections. Wendy finds her identity in relationship, particularly with significant partners.

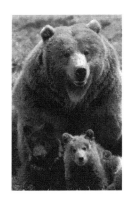

The desire to reach goals never motivated Wendy to make exercise part of her daily life. The best strategy for Wendy would be to work out with someone who meant something special to her – like her boyfriend. This simple connection makes all the difference in the world. And what would be the ideal workout for her to do? Anything – as long as she and her boyfriend did it together.

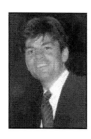 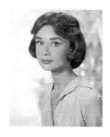

- Psycho-physio profile: The Thinker; ectomorphic, faster metabolism; sensitive to cold; logical, appears unemotional; linear movement patterns; "smart" competitors
- Intrinsic Motivator: Strong Standards, "doing the right thing."
- Inner Destabilizer: Overworking
- Reaction: Burnout
- Compatible Workouts: T'ai Chi Ch'uan, weight training, hatha yoga, Pilates, cycling

Autumn – The Fox

The **Autumn** type is characterized by their love of values, and their high degree of personal integrity. They are deep thinkers, whose thoughts may also be quick and sharp (compare them to deep, slow thinkers, like Winter). Think of them as "witty." Autumn types are characteristically logical and linear.

Autumn types tend to internalize their emotions -- or perhaps it is better said that they have the ability to put their emotions to one side. Often others may interpret this as being aloof, or even "unemotional." In fact, Autumn types feel their emotions quite deeply, but they have the ability to keep their emotions in perspective, and not let them overly cloud a central issue.

Physically, Autumn types to be smaller boned, with a more compact musculature, and a characteristically upright posture. Their movements -- like their thoughts -- tend to be quicker, more precise and commonly linear. They have an aversion to cold and often times to wind. Autumn types typically have a high tolerance for discomfort, and so they often run the risk of overworking.

The **Autumn** type's most powerful intrinsic motivator is their sense of standards, which manifests itself as a strong sense of morality, and a desire to " do the right thing." Autumns are characteristically very logical, so exercise education often works well as a motivator for them. Becoming fit, well or healthy is the right thing to do, both for themselves and for their family. If they work with a coach or trainer for their initial period of exercise -- the first three weeks for example – Au exercise habit. They are then more likely to religiously follow their exercise routine -- almost as if inertia was keeping them from stopping. Now it will take a powerful outside force to get the Autumn to stop working out.

On the other side of this coin, however, is the potential for Autumn types to become obsessive/compulsive about their workouts. They are susceptible to over-training, because they forget that the body needs to rest. When they're on a roll, Autumns have a high tolerance for discomfort, and so may ignore pain or other warning signals. Autumn types need an opportunity to get" out of their heads," find calm, and have fun. Workouts which may balance the Autumn type are activities like T'ai Chi Ch'uan, swimming and ballroom dancing.

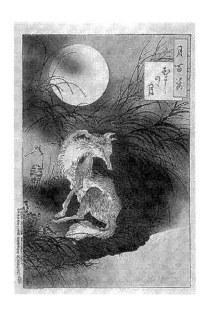

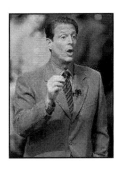

- ➢ Psycho-physio profileStrategist; endomorphic, with strong musculature; systemic thinkers, need to be early risers; appears aloof
- ➢ Intrinsic Motivator: Seeing the Big Picture
- ➢ Inner Destabilizer: Decreasing physical activity
- ➢ Reaction: Surprise, anger, self-criticism, denial
- ➢ Compatible Workouts: body-building, ashtanga yoga, martial arts, cardio-kickboxing, tennis, golf, swimming, Chen style T'ai Chi Ch'uan

Winter – The Ox

The **Winter** type is characterized by their ability to see the big picture. They tend to be larger boned endomorphic, often sturdy and muscular, but may tend toward a slower metabolism. Early mornings make the best times for Winters to exercise. Like Indian Summer types, if they get up and get active upon first awakening, they will do well and feel energetic for the rest of the day. On the other hand, if they lay in bed or fall back asleep, they may have trouble fully waking up, and may feel sluggish for the rest of the day.

The Winter type has a great sense of they way things are connected in time. They see not only the present situation as it is, but also what has been its history and what will be its likely future. They are "Holistic thinkers," which means they see things from a synergistic, systems point of view. They take their time gathering information, and once they see the whole picture, then they act decisively.

Winters are patient listeners -- up to a point. They listen to gather information, not necessarily to understand another's emotions the way Indian Summers do. For some people, the Winter's inwardly directed attention may appear aloof, even cynical. In truth, however, the Winter type is more likely processing information, keeping what is relevant, throwing out what is superfluous, and creating strategies for setting and attaining goals.

Both **Winter and Indian Summer** types have similar physical characteristics, and share certain mental traits as well. Both types tend toward a slower metabolism. Especially as they get older, their "inner fires" tend to burn down to the embers. They settle into themselves, like bears getting ready for hibernation. For this reason, Indian Summers and Winters need constant, regular stimulation. Change and challenge is healthy for them. Tennis, fencing, swimming or martial arts are all recommended. If an individual were drawn to Classical mind/body disciplines, then the more vigorous styles like Chen T'ai Chi or Ashtanga yoga would be more beneficial.

Indian Summers and Winters have different personality types, however, and different intrinsic motivators. Indian Summers have a strong emotional component to their personalities, while Winters typically have a strong mental component. Both are systemic, Holistic thinkers, but it is Winter who is more concerned about "the big picture." He wants to know, "What will this workout do for me? How will it fit in with everything else I'm doing?" A logical approach, with a good schedule is very persuasive to the Winter type. On the other hand, the Indian Summer is highly motivated by the connection to a group -- a family, company, church or significant other. Indian Summers will be interested in just about any activity, as long as they do it with some other people who are important in their lives.

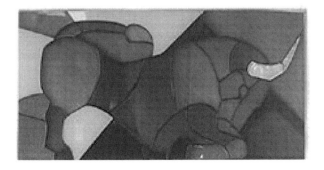

Take the Test -- Discover your own BodyMind Season

In each of the following section, score each statement by rating it on a scale of 1-5. 1="This must be someone else." 5="That's me to a T!" When you have finished scoring all five sections, look for the section with the highest score, and compare it to the key at the end of the test. Have fun!

Section A.
1. __4__ I like things to be well defined, neat and tidy, and I do well with discipline.
2. __3__ I tend to be on the thinner side, and if I do gain weight, I can lose it easily.
3. __4__ I feel loved the most when I'm given constant words of affirmation.
4. __4__ I try to live according to reason and logical principles.
5. __5__ I admire beauty and refinement, and enjoy logical principles.
6. __5__ I like to choose my words carefully.
7. __1__ I often get cold hands or feet, and sometimes dry skin or hair.
8. __2__ I tend to move quickly, but precisely and meticulously.
9. __2__ I may sometimes seem too formal and distant, even self-righteous.
10. __4__ Intense emotions sometimes make me withdraw – but that doesn't mean I don't have feelings.

Total: __34__

Section B.
1. __3__ I savor excitement and spontaneity and I delight in intimacy.
2. __3__ I am keenly intuitive and passionately empathetic.
3. __4__ I believe in the power of charisma and desire.
4. __3__ I feel the most loved when someone gives me special gifts.
5. __1__ I like to be the life of the party.
6. __1__ Being emotionally stressed makes me tired, or sometimes cranky.
7. __2__ I like to be hot, vibrant and bright.
8. __2__ I usually have a good shape and physique, but if I'm not careful I an gain weight in all the wrong places.
9. __2__ I have a fairly rapid pulse.
10. __2__ When I'm stressed, I look for something to make me feel better: a drink, a smoke, some chocolate – or even going to the movies.

Total: __23__

89

Section C.
1. __4__ I love a challenge, and like to push the edges of the envelope.
2. __3__ I do well under pressure.
3. __3__ I admire speed, novelty and skill.
4. __2__ I'm usually good at sports.
5. __4__ I like being a winner – I strive to be first and best.
6. __3__ I'm a take-charge kind of person.
7. __3__ I hate taking "no" for an answer.
8. __4__ I feel the most loved when I get physical attention from another person.
9. __4__ I do well when I set specific goals for myself.
10. __4__ I drink coffee regularly.

Total: __34__

Section D.
1. __5__ There is nothing more comforting than having your family around you.
2. __4__ I don't mind being in charge, as long as I don't have to be in the spotlight.
3. __5__ I am agreeable and accommodating.
4. __5__ I believe in peace, harmony and togetherness.
5. __5__ I believe people can always find a way to get along – if they try.
6. __4__ Even when I get very sad, I take care not to show it.
7. __5__ I feel the most loved when someone spends quality time with me.
8. __3__ If I'm not careful, I tend to be lethargic.
9. __1__ I am a large-boned person, and can gain weight fairly easily.
10. __1__ I sometimes form unreasonable expectations, which can lead to disappointment.

Total: __38__

Section E.
1. __4__ I'm good at creating the strategies that make things happen.
2. __5__ I tend to be introspective, self-contained and self-sufficient.
3. __3__ I have a penetrating and critical mind, and I like to examine things closely.
4. __1__ I am a big-boned person, but I was quite active when I was young.
5. __3__ I like to be behind the scenes, acting anonymously.
6. __3__ I tend to live in my head.
7. __4__ I value knowledge and understanding.
8. __2__ I feel the most loved when someone does important things for me – "acts of service."
9. __4__ I'm not comfortable when things are unorganized, inefficient or haphazard.
10. __5__ I'm the kind of person who says, 'Look before you leap."
Total: __34__

Record your scores: A __34__ B __23__ C __34__ D __38__ E __34__

(Here's your Key: A=Autumn; B=Summer; C=Spring, D= Indian Summer; E=Winter)

By the way, you can also take this test for free online at
www.thewellnessevolution.com.

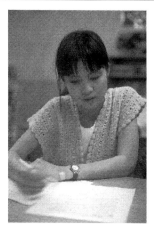

A Final Thought

Every new experience is by definition a situation of stress. Stress, as we know, triggers people to retreat in the extremes of their BodyMind type. If your new experience matches your BodyMind dynamics, then you remember the experience in a positive way. But if the experience is a odds with your BodyMind Season, then you will usually remember it negatively. So, if we know that, why would we choose experiences that would create a bad memory of an activity, when we could just as easily choose an experience that would create a good memory.

Two final things to remember about the Five-Season System: First, it is a model-- a map of the territory, not the territory itself. It's not meant to assume every detail, only the general terrain. Secondly, the typology is a "system," not an artifact. It is a series of "if-thens," not a concrete "this is it."

Although in the Conventional fitness model, trainers do assess people individually, they do it based on a tacit assumption that all people experience their bodies in the same way. For example, many trainers individually assess their clients, and look for specific individual postural distortions, muscle weaknesses or imbalances, and loss of range of motion. But rarely do those same trainers stop to investigate why that individual exhibits the conditions the trainer discovers. Why these particular conditions, at this time, in this person? Moreover, as trainers distinguish those conditions, they typically view them as something to be fixed, with a set of protocols (i.e. workouts or therapies) that match the condition, rather than the person.

The most important thing about using the principle of diversity and the BodyMind typology is that without them, any assessment or programming protocol would either be too generic or would have no predictability of being repeatable – in other words, it would have no scientific validity. As we'll see in the next chapter, in order to unleash the experience of power, freedom and flow in your life, you have to discover what it is that covers it up.

Chapter III: Elements

The gift of the third chapter, Elements, is *choice*. This chapter explains the elements that make up the Holistic approach. More than anything else, I want to show you a universe of options and possibilities you may have never considered. Open this gift, and I hope to hear you say, "I now see choices for my life and my health I never knew I had before."

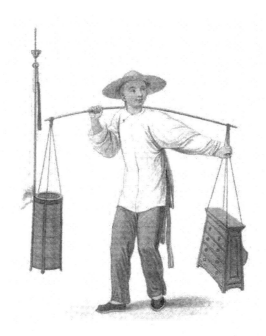

In Chapter I, we began to consider a way of treating the body, mind and Spirit in a way that would give us a different experience of life than the one we often have. Specifically, we proposed that goal of the holistic approach to fitness, wellness and health was to experience being perfect and complete, with Power, Freedom and Flow coursing through our lives every minute of every day. This is what I call a *soulful* experience of life – because soul is the name we give to our authentic inner Self.

In this chapter, we'll begin to explore the distinctions, concepts and practices of the Holistic approach. Distinctions define and clarify our speech, and make our conversation more powerful and effective. For example, in our current physical culture, we do not typically consider that fitness, wellness and health do not mean the same thing. If we did, we might be more powerful in the way we make choices about how we exercise, eat, or deal with stress. As we learn to make more powerful and informed choices, we may find that the common health practices of physical activity, good nutrition and stress management, can actually be irresistibly fun as well as effective.

The principles underlying any one realm of the Holistic approach guide every realm. For example, the principles that underlie the physical realm also apply to the mental and Spiritual realms, and whatever I say about physical activity also will apply to diet and stress management. In the physical realm, for example, the Holistic approach is concerned with physical activity, nutrition and stress management. In the mental realm, the Holistic approach is concerned with both emotional and intellectual thought and the development of the will power. In the Spiritual realm, the Holistic approach is concerned with an individual's sense of there being something greater than oneself, and with the discovery of deeper levels of consciousness.

Happiness

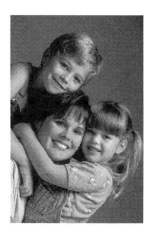

I've kept a journal for more than 20 years, and I write in it almost every day. So many times I've written in my journals the complaints of my love affairs gone wrong, or of my career disappointments. "Where is the joy?" I wonder, reading the entries from years past. If some historian in the future were to read my diary, would he or she conclude that I was a morose, melancholy man who was frustrated and unhappy with life?

"But no!" my ghost would cry. I am filled with an exuberance of life. I laugh with children and wink at grandmothers. I wink at grand*fathers*. I am an eternal romantic, and no matter how many times I've loved and lost, I am ready to love again.

But the greatest joy I've ever had was being a nice person. It's so simple it sounds simple-minded. But the truth — my truth — is that once I gave myself permission to be nice, my whole experience of life shifted. Like Elwood P. Dowd (the main character in the movie *Harvey*) said, "In this life one can either be oh so smart, or oh so pleasant." And like Elwood, for years I was smart. I too recommend pleasant. What pleasant meant for me was appreciating the inner beauty of every person I meet. The opportunity to contribute to another's life is supremely fulfilling.

What is it that makes one enduringly happy? The Epicureans of ancient Greece proposed that happiness is the highest good, and therefore whatever causes our happiness is also therefore good. The Dalai Lama says there is an art to happiness. He says, "Happiness can be achieved through the systematic training of our hearts and minds, through re-shaping our attitudes and outlook." Happiness, in other words, is all in our heads. I guess it's just as your mother always said: "Change that attitude, Bud."

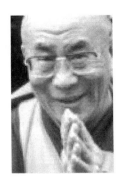

Consider, however, that happiness, like health, is a naturally occurring experience. Your happiness is inside you all the time, itching to get out. Your happiness is at this very moment dancing from foot to foot, the way kids do waiting in line at the ice cream truck. Not patiently at all.

But just like health, our happiness slams headlong into our masks and compensations. Happiness cannot last in an environment of inauthenticity. Oh, we may experience moments of pleasure – even ecstasy – but it doesn't endure. And the disappearance of those moments leaves us like the Flying Dutchman, forever seeking an elusive bliss. On the other hand – and this is the million-dollar secret – when we remove our masks, and our compensations disappear, our happiness appears, sighing, "I've been here the whole time."

Health and happiness go together. How can you be truly happy without your health? And who would even care if they were healthy or not if they weren't happy?

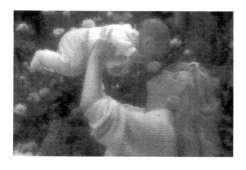

Balance

> To the ordinary being, others often require tolerance.
> To the highly evolved being, there is no such thing as tolerance, because there is no such thing as other.
> She has given up all ideas of individuality and extended her goodwill without prejudice in every direction.
> Never hating, never resisting, never contesting, she is simply always learning and being.
>
> Loving, hating, having expectations: all these are attachments.
> Attachment prevents the growth of one's true being.
> Therefore the integral being is attached to nothing and can relate to everyone with an unstructured attitude.
> Because of this, her very existence benefits all things.
> -- Lao Tzu, *The Hua Hu Ching*

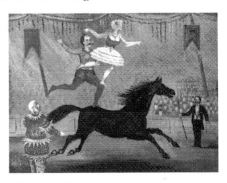

The first principle of the Holistic approach is the Principle of **Balance.** Consider that inherent in the concept of being perfect and complete is the trait of being balanced and in harmony. In fact, the body's natural systems of healing and longevity depend upon this balance and harmony. An internal environment that is out of balance is what leads to dysfunction and disease. Being out of balance also skews your perspective. It's hard to move gracefully from point to point (or from choice to choice) when we're out of balance. On the other hand, being in balance is a position from which you can do anything. Bottom line: balance just "feels" better.

Everything we do in life is either a step towards balance or a step away from balance. The Holistic approach is to make choices in life that restore and/or promote balance, because the farther away from balance we stray, the more perfection is concealed; the closer to balance we return, the more our completeness is revealed.

According to the great yogi B.K.S. Iyengar, "The supreme adventure in a man's life is his journey back to his Creator. To reach the goal he needs well developed and coordinated functioning of his body, senses, mind, reason and Self. If the effort is not coordinated, he fails in his adventure." In other words, balance and harmony are essential to the sense of fulfillment in life. Each of us grows up differently, and often with the body, mind and Spirit uncoordinated, or *out* of balance. Your mind may be stronger than your body, or perhaps your body is stronger than your mind and spirit. But what happens when these three sides of yourself are out of balance?

(What would the Scarecrow and the Tin Man be like without the Cowardly Lion?) Think about it: body worshipped without mind is often brutish and vain, and body without spirit is frivolous. A mind developed without a healthy body is frail and short-lived, while a mind without spirit is insensitive. Finally, even a great spirit without a body is too ephemeral, and spirit without mind is chaotic.

The Wellness Triangle

One of the first places to look to see if you're living life in balance is the "Wellness Triangle." These are the three intersecting sets of lifestyle habits that lead to Wellness: physical activity, stress management and nutrition. Every experience of life falls into one of these categories. For example, nutrition includes everything that you ingest and digest – including air, water, food (of course), alcohol, drugs (recreational or prescription), cigarette smoke (yours or second hand), candy and so on. Stress management includes all the experiences of managing your inner and outer relationships, and your inner and outer conflicts and confrontations. It includes how you prepare for and then handle the subtle and unexpected stressors of daily life, like traffic, noise or weather. Even things that are done to promote wellness, like changing diet or exercising are stressors, and stress management is how you deal with them. By "stress management" we also refer to one's spiritual side – one's sense of the Divine, or even simply seeing that the world is bigger than oneself. Finally, physical activity is all the ways in which you move your body – or avoid moving. This would include what we call exercise, recreation, sports and dance – but also how we sit, stand, and sleep; the safety and ergonomics of our work, etc. It is how we center and orient ourselves in our physical world, and move around in it.

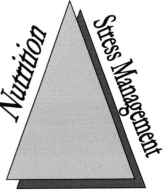

Integrity, Compassion and Synergy

Integrity is often interpreted as meaning adherence to a high moral standard – but that's not the original intent of the word. Integrity comes from the Middle English *integrite*, a word itself derived from the Latin words *integritas*, meaning soundness, and *integer*, meaning whole and complete. Nothing is "missing" in a state of integrity; but more than that, nothing is "leaking out." In ships, for example, the word *integrity* is used to describe the quality of being leak-proof, as in "water-tight integrity." Integrity means being true to your word, so that others' trust in you doesn't leak away. Integrity means acting in a way in alignment with being perfect and complete. Integrity means conserving, rather than consuming, your vital life energy. When Integrity is present, you experience **Power** in your life.

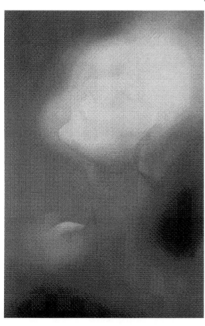

Compassion means remembering everyone is perfect – including you. Acceptance, not judgment or blame, resolves conflict and treats imbalances. At the heart of the Holistic approach is the philosophy that our deepest, truest nature is to be perfect and complete; therefore, we can be patient and kind with others and ourselves. The experience of suffering is something the entire world shares – physical aches and pains, disease and early mortality, the destructive emotions of anger, craving and fear. In fact, the original meaning of compassion is "to suffer together." It's human to experience suffering in life. Consider that suffering arises when our inherent perfection is concealed, and we embrace the illusion that there is something wrong that needs to be fixed or improved. Of course that suffering *feels* real – that's the point. Compassion is being firm in your unconditional acceptance, and steadfast in the stand that life is perfect and whole, even in the face of suffering. When Compassion is present, you experience **Freedom** in your life.

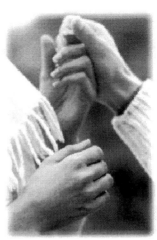

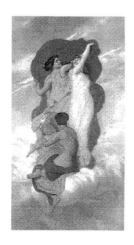

Synergy means the conscious and continuous interweaving of body, mind and Spirit. No part of the self can be isolated from another, because no part exists without the others. Synergy is the ability of all parts to work together, creating a whole that is greater than the sum of its parts. Stress is a barrier to synergy, dissociation is a barrier to synergy, reductionism is also a barrier to synergy. Also some methodologies may not work well together, and thereby prevent synergy. When Synergy is present, you experience **Flow** in your life.

Sensation/Perception Cycle

Sensation is what we feel – the literal information that comes from our five senses of sight, sound, touch, taste and smell, and from our other sensory nerves, including the proprioceptors (for coordination and balance) and nociceptors (for pain). Consider, however, that all this raw data must eventually be processed and interpreted by the brain. This is what we call "perception." Perception by definition is a story or explanation of our sensations. For example, we can interpret the same sensation either as discomfort and pain, or as stimulation and exhilaration. Some people love roller coasters; some people hate them.

As human beings, we actually have the ability to shift our perceptions at will. For example, there are many techniques for managing, lessening or disappearing pain sensations. Martial artists and women preparing for natural childbirth use these techniques. These individuals have taken a sensation and created a positive or neutral interpretation, or perception. By the same token, some people create a negative association with particular sensations. This perception now induces or increases the feeling of pain or fear whenever that sensation is felt.

When a sensation is felt, the brain immediately creates a perception, or explanation of what's going on. Now, whenever a similar environment or circumstance is detected, the body expects a repeat of the initial sensation. Sure enough, when that sensation occurs, it seems like a reinforcement of the original perception. Now a sensation/perception cycle has been initiated. If the perception is one of pain or danger, then the body reacts naturally to protect itself. The accumulation of these reactions – twitches, hitches, hunches, turnouts etc. – creates a pattern of compensatory movements that become ingrained in the body. Now the body automatically and unconsciously holds a posture and a movement pattern that is a result of the sensation/perception cycle.

Spontaneous Healing

At this point you may be asking, "So how does the Holistic approach actually work? How can I liberate myself from the patterns and compensations of my past?" The principle of **Spontaneous Healing** says that given the right conditions, or access beneath the mask, the body (as well as the mind or Spirit) *will renew itself.* The true meaning of the word, "heal," in fact means, "to make whole." Healing is the process of restoring your *experience* of being perfect, whole and complete. In other words, the only reason we are ever sick, in pain or injured is because something stands between us and our inner healer: our masks. All we need to do, therefore, is find a way to get underneath the mask, interrupt the pattern of compensation, and remove the barriers, and our innate wholeness will be revealed.

But how, we might ask, does that really happen? How does healing take place in a paradigm in which there's no fixing or improving? Simply put, part of the miraculous perfection of being human is that the body (as well as the mind or Spirit) has everything it needs to carry out a spontaneous re-creation of any damaged part. Like the salamander that can slough off his tail and then grow a new one, we have within every cell of our bodies the complete DNA code to re-form the rest of the body.

When we recover from an injury or recuperate from an illness, it is because our own natural systems of healing made it so. Drugs, surgery, acupuncture or laying on of hands may have been involved – but the most any of these types of treatments can do is help create the conditions under which the body healed itself.

Unmasking the BodyMind

Discovery is the process of distinguishing what might be concealing an individual's perfection. In this chapter we're going to take a look specifically at how we can recognize and understand the masks we've created by literally looking at ourselves in a mirror. What kinds of masks have we created, and what do they look like on us? We need to understand the masks so that we can understand how to get underneath them.

Let's look at three types of masks, using a model developed by master life coach Tom Stone called the "Core Dynamics." For our purposes, the Core Dynamics model has been adapted to allow us to see those masks at play on the physical plane. In addition to the three deep inner dynamic, there are also common symptoms associated with each mask. For example, one of the symptoms of the second mask, "Looking for Yourself Where You're Not," is the habit of mistaking need for love.

The first mask is the mask of Trying to Force an Outcome. Ramming square pegs into the round holes of your life is forcing an outcome. We frequently see this mask when we use too much physical or emotional strength, or the position of authority, to dominate others – or to avoid being dominated by them.

Mental/emotional symptoms of the inner dynamics*:

(According to Tom Stone's Core Dynamics model)

- Manufacturing interpretations
- Excluding other perspectives
- Over-reacting to circumstances

The second mask is the mask of Looking for Yourself Where You Are Not. A common example of this is looking for personal validation in the approval of others, even though true self-esteem is independent of anyone's opinion. As Tom Stone says, "What other people think of me is none of my business."

Mental/emotional symptoms of the inner dynamics:

- Resisting change
- Mistaking need for love
- Limiting self-expression

The third mask is the mask of Resisting Feeling Things Fully. For many of us, the impact of emotions feels frighteningly intense – even physically painful. Built into our human dna is an instinct for "harm-avoidance," and in most of us this shows up as a physical reaction known as the "startle reflex." When we hear an unexpected loud noise (car backfire, for example) we flinch, blink our eyes, and hunch our shoulders in anticipation of the pain that may follow the thunderclap. Internally, we shut down in the same way to avoid hearing the messages of our emotions and instincts. When we resist feeling things fully, however, we also cut ourselves off from the messages of our own intuition.

Mental/emotional symptoms of the inner dynamics:

- Being judgmental
- Ignoring your intuition
- Avoiding the present

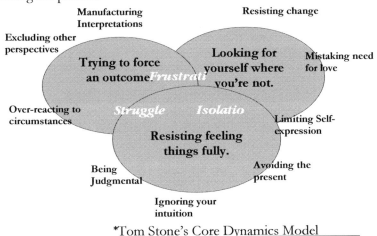

*Tom Stone's Core Dynamics Model

The thing to remember is that we don't usually see masks as masks. What we see are symptoms, like physical pain, chronic injury, depression, weak muscles, poor posture, eating disorders, allergies, chronic disease, relationship breakdowns, or inability to lose/gain weight at will. Just below the symptoms, however, we'll discover patterns -- patterns of habit, patterns of movement, patterns of structure. On a physical level, we often see these patterns manifest themselves as postural distortions, or muscle imbalances. What causes these patterns to begin to form in the first place might be injury, poor posture, dysfunctional movement patterns, or any number of psychogenic causes. Note that all of these can be boiled down to one thing: disconnection. Disconnection, also known as dissociation, leads to a postural distortion. Postural distortion causes a compensation to form. Now the compensations themselves begin to cause greater disconnects, leading to greater distortion, and so on in a vicious cycle.

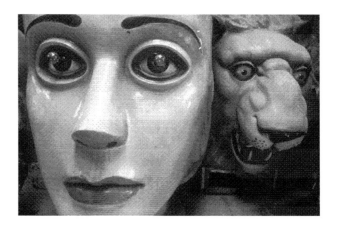

My girlfriend Michelle broke her tailbone running track in high school. By the time I met her, she had a condition of chronic back pain and sciatica that sometimes left her unable to move or even get out of bed. She would try to bear the discomfort for as long as she could, and then get an emergency appointment with her chiropractor to relieve the pain. Sometimes, the chiropractor said, her spine was so locked up that he couldn't get her back to adjust. X-rays revealed that she had developed scoliosis, a side-to-side curvature of the spine. She also had developed a tilted and rotated pelvis – specifically a posterior rotation on her right side. She asked the doctor what she could do about it. He said, "Nothing."

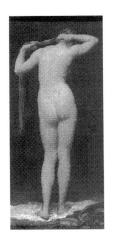

Breaking your tailbone hurts a lot, and for a while your body has to shut down that area while it heals. It swells, which is one way that the body provides a cushion, like an air brace, around the broken bones. The swelling also indicates an increased flow of blood and lymph into the area, bringing oxygen, nutrients and white blood cells to the injury, and carrying away lactic acids and damaged cells. The tenderness of a swollen area is also a natural "keep away" message, and if in addition your doctor gives you any pain pills, then you can really start to disconnect from that area.

Meanwhile, Michelle still had to move. Her body began to compensate, recruiting other muscles to keep her lower back straight and to swing her leg in its socket. Her body was trying to create new functionality. Unfortunately, these compensations were actually a distortion of the way her body was meant to function, and the longer those compensations remained in effect, the more they became permanent distortions.

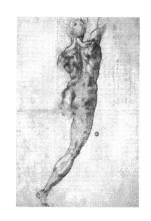

In a way, you could say that her body "forgot" the way it was designed to stand and move. You see, ideally, the muscles of the body are combined in groups, each muscle in the group exerting a force on the bones to hold them in place in perfectly neutral alignment. Each muscle in the group has an ideal length when at rest, and exerts an ideal amount of tension on the bone. The cumulative tension contributed by each of the muscles in the group is called the "force couple." When Michelle's bones – the internal scaffolding of her body – were moved out of alignment, then some of her muscles got stretched and loose and some of her muscles got short and tight. The force couple was altered. This is what happens when your body creates a physical compensation in an attempt to gain greater functionality. Over time, your body gets used to this altered force couple, and your bones are pulled toward the shorter, tighter muscles.

The Six Universal Compensations

As I said earlier, we rarely see the core dynamics at work in a person's life immediately. What we usually see are the symptoms of those dynamics, and those symptoms combine to make patterns – patterns of movement, behavior, action and reaction.

Each of us has a unique life history that shows up in our bodies, thoughts, emotions and Spirit. The nuances of our life experiences can combine in an infinite variety of symptoms and compensation patterns. At the same time, our lives unfold on a common stage called 'being human," and over the years I have observed that some patterns appear over and over. I call these "The Six Universal Compensations that Mask Wholeness." I call them "universal" because my experience is that people will tend to react to stress the same way, time after time regardless of the situation -- unless of course, they consciously develop the skills to react differently.

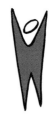

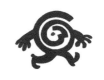

Heaviness

The first class of symptoms called is "Heaviness," which describes what happens when you use the body as nothing more than a thing – a tool to force an outcome. Many people whose work is strenuous physical labor use Heaviness as a way of pushing themselves to accomplish more. Athletes develop Heaviness patterns to make their bodies perform at high levels.

How that looks in the body is often muscle imbalances, where on one side of the body muscles are stronger and tighter, while on the other side, the same muscles of weak and overstretched. There's also often a hypertonicity in the muscles, which means that there is an unnatural state of being flexed all the time. Often we'll find muscles that twitch, or have a very low threshold of activation.

In life, Heaviness can manifest as a person who uses too much muscular or emotional force to control life or to resist being controlled. For example, the partner, parent or boss who use intimidation or interrogation to dominate the relationship is using Heaviness.

Common Physical Symptoms:

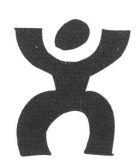

- Over-activation of muscles
- Hypertonicity
- Muscle Imbalances

Lightness

The second class of symptoms is "Lightness," the phenomenon of beginning to lose contact with your physical nature -- usually because you have stopped "listening" to your body. In this case, reactions may be a result of assuming you know what your body is saying instead of honestly reacting to your body. Lightness also shows up in the way we relate or communicate to other people. If you've ever thought to yourself, "I won't even bother asking... I know what she's going to say," then you've experienced Lightness.

Common Physical Symptoms:

- Under-activation
- Poor proprioception

Breaking

After Lightness comes "Breaking." This is when you completely lose contact with your physicality. Two things occur when this happens. First, your body cannot get enough information from your central nervous system to nurture, stimulate or otherwise communicate with you. Second, you don't have enough connection to your body to sense when it is in transition. Breaking is a total disconnection. But Breaking can also be subtler. If you find yourself retreating within, and closing down emotionally in reaction to stress, then even if you are still physically present you have still lost contact with yourself.

Common Physical Symptoms:
- Dissociation
- Atrophy

Stiffness

The fourth class of symptoms is called "Stiffness." Stiffness is the lack of flexibility around either the center or the joints of the body. There is a familiar technique in playing the T'ai Chi game of Push Hands: if you can maneuver the other person into a position where they cannot turn the waist or relax their joints then you can easily push them over. You've found out where they are Stiff.

In the body, Stiffness is marked by a lack of flexibility, and sometimes not being very good at feeling where your body is in space. Prejudice and fear-based thought are examples of Stiffness. They bring you to a position where you feel you cannot bend any more -- that's as far as you can go. But you may find that if you relax your attachment to one particular point of view, your center will loosen up and you will be a much more emotionally flexible person.

Common Physical Symptoms:
- Inflexibility
- Lack of proprioception

Misdirection

The fifth most common reason for losing your balance in a relationship is "Misdirection." This is the characteristic of being led farther and farther away from your center. Misdirection is a favorite avoidance technique -- teenagers are masters at it. Characteristic signs of misdirection are altered force couples. This is when muscles are pulling on the joint and bones in an altered, dysfunctional or inefficient pattern. This is what happens when the normal angle of pull has been changed for some reason.

Common Physical Symptoms:

- Inactive core
- Altered force couple
- Synergistic dominance
- Weight Shifting

Monotony

The last in our list of the most common causes of conflict is "Monotony." Remember, yin and yang combine in an endless pattern of possible combinations. Always reacting in the same way is not allowing for many of these possibilities. This is Monotony. In the body, this can look like always eating the same foods, or always preparing them in the same way.

One of the more interesting manifestations of physical Monotony are repetitive or monoplanar movements. As a Wellness Coach, when I analyze how people move through three-dimensional space I break down their movements into three different directions, or planes, of motion. For example, when you move directly forward and backward, this is called moving in the saggital plane. Moving directly side to side is moving in the frontal plane, and when you turn side to side is moving in the transverse plane.

Ideally, we use all three planes of movement to gracefully move through space (and life). Often, however, I meet clients who have developed a pattern of moving predominantly in only one or two planes. They seem to move a little like robots, repeat the same pattern of walking, carrying – even speaking – in the same way over and over. Their whole lives seem to be played out in the same plane, as thought they lived in two-dimensional world.

Common Physical Symptoms:
- Monoplanar movement
- Extreme linearity

A Final Thought

I began writing this book as an expression of my work as a teacher, fitness expert, coach and healer. When I began working in the fitness industry more than 20 years ago, it didn't seem to me that we had a "philosophy of fitness." My education seemed to be mostly concerned with programs, choreography and technique. That seemed incomplete, somehow. I felt that it was just as important to know *why* we do what we do as fitness professionals as to know how to do it.

I am so grateful to be part of the fitness industry, but it is clear that the industry has a different focus than either wellness or health. The center of attention in physical fitness education for the last 25 years has been on developing mechanical techniques: pumping iron to build bigger, stronger bodies; dancing and running to develop greater aerobic capacities; and stretching to improve mobility. In other words, we have spent our efforts looking for the best ways to work harder, mechanically.

But mechanical exercise can overly stress the body, wasting vital energy and even creating disease. Moreover, mechanical (Conventional) exercise uses only half of the brain -- the left side; the analytical side, the side that looks at "parts" and tells you only how to move. It is the right side of the brain that calls upon the imagination, and looks at the poetry and metaphors our movements.

The holistic approach is a change in the philosophy of fitness to one of fully mindful exercise. Mindful exercise uses the whole brain. It integrates the right side function -- the creative, non-linear, holistic side, the side which houses that often un-tapped potential for limitless power and excellent performance -- with the analytical "how-to" left brain.

In T'ai Chi and yoga, my first disciplines, philosophy and movement are Siamese twins. In these systems we learn that everything we do – from sleeping and eating to working or working out – is fueled by our intrinsic life force. The Chinese call intrinsic energy qi, the Japanese say ki, the ancient Hindus called it kundalini. By whatever name we call it, there is within each of us the vital spirit that is life. It fuels everything we do: our thoughts, our feelings, and of course our movements. And like a fuel, eventually the vital life energy runs out. Our motors cease to turn, our life ends. The question is: how fuel-efficient is your activity? Do you scream up and down the road, pushing yourself to the red line just to show off between stoplights? Or do you know how to elegantly purr down the highway, looking good, running smooth and rolling on and on and on?

Several years ago, I was asked to become a member of the Mind/Body Exercise committee for the world's largest health and fitness organization, IDEA. One of the first things I wanted to do as a new committee member was to help create a more succinct and comprehensive definition for Mind/Body exercise. (Believe it or not, at the time we really did not know how to define this "new" genre of fitness.)

I was motivated partly by the desire to find a way to prove to Conventional fitness that T'ai Chi Ch'uan was a superior workout. I had been focusing on studying, teaching and promoting T'ai Chi for 20 years, I was not used to looking for the good points in anything else. I had developed a pattern of thinking that there was something wrong with any system that didn't include of philosophy of energy. And of course, if I could come up with a great new definition of mind/body fitness, based on the teachings of T'ai Chi Ch'uan, it would "fix" the whole fitness industry.

But in the process of writing a new definition, I had a personal breakthrough in my understanding of Holistic exercise. I realized that regardless of how many benefits T'ai Chi has to offer, T'ai Chi is not necessarily "better" than any other form of exercise. "Better" is a subjective quality, and every person must make their own choice as to what is best for them at any particular time in their lives. I began to see that no particular exercise was magically or inherently better than any other, because the magic lies in the way the work is done – and even more importantly, *who* is doing the work. It finally dawned on me that I was myself operating from a very conventional point of view: that something was wrong that needed to be fixed or improved. I had just substituted holistic-sounding exercises for the more common Conventional ones.

I started by attempting to find a way to explain why T'ai Chi was different than the other workouts. I knew intuitively that though we might call, say, "Mind/Body Power Lifting" a "mind/body exercise," you couldn't say that was in the same category as T'ai Chi Ch'uan and Hatha yoga. But the more I studied the various other mind/body workouts, the more I came to understand that they all echoed, in one way or another, the principles that were what I had learned as the fundamentals of T'ai Chi Ch'uan.

The truth, I realized, was that a wide range of physical activity could be holistic. When the body moves in the rhythms of skiing, surfing, step aerobics, cycling, running, T'ai Chi, yoga, dancing, or whatever, something inside you intuitively recognizes the depth and value of this movement and responds. It gets "exercised." It grows stronger, and begins to show its insights at other moments of life, looking for more ways to connect to other people, to the natural environment, and even to the Divine.

At last I was in able to break free of my attachment to thinking of T'ai Chi as the "best" exercise. All exercise can be holistic. Even the most conventional workouts are in some sense "mind/body." Weightlifters, at the very least, "think" about which weight they're going to pick up. In an aerobics class, you try to recognize the pattern of the teachers' movements.

The elements of the Holistic approach are more concerned with context than with content. Even yoga postures can be performed mindlessly and without any meditative attitude, while power lifting can be done like a prayer, like a meditation, integrating body, mind and Spirit.

To be human is to tread a path on which every step is another crossroad. Every moment of our lives we are given an opportunity to choose how we think, act or feel. But how do we make those choices? How, in fact, do we even understand the choices we are given? Underlying the Holistic approach is a set of principles that starts to create the context and the structure for our choice making.

As long as we focus on the mechanics of our lives then our choices appear limited. We focus on what is available, rather than what is possible. But a philosophy of life that considers one's "being" as well as one's "doing" opens the opportunity for the exercise of the free will, and frees us to make limitless choices at the crossroads of life.

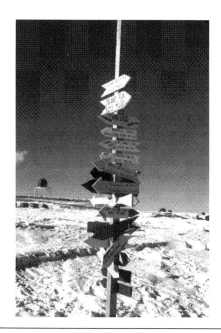

Desideratum #1: Fitness, Wellness & Health

A desideratum is something desired as essential or needed. You may have noticed that throughout this book, I've referred to fitness, wellness and health as separate things. This is a contrast to the Conventional approach, which typically treats fitness, wellness and health as interchangeable. Like the longer chapters in this book, this mini-chapter is also a gift. Open it, and I hope to hear you say, "I can now see how making a clear distinction between fitness, wellness and health allows me to guide my actions toward my true desires."

Fitness, Wellness and Health

The Holistic approach recognizes that people are searching for a soulful experience of life in many different ways. Often we don't really know how to pinpoint or articulate what we want because we don't know how to distinguish – that is, recognize and speak about – what is missing in our lives. In America's physical culture the concepts of fitness, wellness and health get collapsed all together, as though they meant the same thing. You may have noticed, for example, that I frequently write these words as a list, rather than just using them interchangeably. In this chapter, we pull these concepts apart. By distinguishing them as separate pursuits, one can make more appropriate choices about the actions we take to uncover our wholeness and perfection.

> *Health is a state of wholeness -- and focuses not just on the body, but on the mind and spirit as well. Whereas fitness is based on an athletic model, and wellness is based on a medical model, health is based on a spiritual model.*

What is important to note is that the Conventional Approach is dominated by the pursuit of Fitness, while the Mind/Body Approach addresses the pursuit of Wellness and Health. This is why we say that the Mind/Body Approach is more complete, because Wellness *includes and transcends* the components of Fitness, and Health *includes and transcends* the components of Wellness.

Fitness

The American Heritage Dictionary Says:

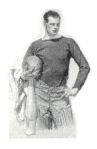

- Fitness: The state or condition of being physically fit, especially as the result of exercise and proper nutrition.
- Fit:
    o To be the proper shape and size
    o To be appropriate
    o To be in conformity
    o To make suitable, adapt

In other words: Based on an athletic model, **Fitness** is the special ability to accomplish physical tasks at an improved level of proficiency, achieved by optimizing the workings of your body through specialized training.

Wellness

The American Heritage Dictionary Says:

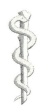

- Wellness: The condition of good physical and mental health, especially maintained by proper diet, exercise and life habits.
- Well:
    o Not ailing, infirm or diseased; healthy
    o Cured or healed, as a wound

In other words: Based on a medical model, **Wellness** is freedom from conditions of mental or physical sickness or pain, and is achieved and maintained through our own lifestyle habits and choices.

Health

The American Heritage Dictionary Says:

- Heal
    - To restore to health or soundness; cure. To set right; repair
    - To restore (a person) to spiritual wholeness.
    - To become whole and sound; return to health
- Whole
    - Containing all components; complete
    - Not divided or disjoined; in one unit.
    - Not wounded, injured or impaired; sound or unhurt.

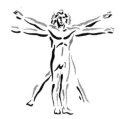

In other words: Based on a spiritual model, **Health** is an experience of being integrated and whole in body, mind, emotions and Spirit.

Fitness

When we use the word, "fitness," we are actually labeling the outward results of physical conditioning through exercise. Fitness is the special ability to accomplish certain physical tasks - to run, jump, swim, climb, fight, hunt, and throw -- at an improved level of proficiency.

This is, in fact, how exercise is valued by most of the West. According to the American Heart Association and the American Cancer Society, the benefits of exercise can be divided into these four components: increasing muscular strength, increasing flexibility, conditioning the heart and lungs, and changing the body's composition so that it has less fat and more muscle - all attributes which contribute to a greater level of physical performance.

Is Fitness for You?

What many people don't know is that many of the standards for measuring fitness were derived by measuring the performance of world-class athletes. These standards assume that fitness is gained by *optimizing* the workings of your body, like the oxygen/nutrient delivery of your cardio-respiratory system, or the activation of your various muscle groups. Researchers typically evaluate aerobic workouts by asking, "Can it increase the *maximum* amount of oxygen uptake into the body?" Studies in nutrition have asked, "Can we determine what diet would create the *maximum* effect of reducing fat in the body?

The Training Effect

Fitness, as we know it in the West, is based on an *athletic* model and is focused on improving performance and appearance. The better your body performs physical tasks and the more endurance and muscular tone you exhibit, the more "fit" you are. Fitness, or athletic, workouts are designed to create a "training effect" in the body -- a semi-permanent change in body composition or physical ability which will lead to improved performance.

To achieve the training effect, athletes follow what is known as the FIT principle, which stands for Frequency, Intensity and Time (or Duration). In a nutshell, an athlete mixes and matches these three factors to stress his body in such a way that it is forced to adapt and change. Athletes and their trainers know, for example, that workouts should be fairly frequent if they want to create results – at least three times a weeks is just about the minimum frequency required to instigate the processes of adaptation in the body.

The Beauty of Fitness

Of course, I don't mean to suggest in any way that fitness is not a good thing. Fitness training can contribute to improved physical abilities, a sense of pride and an improved self-image. Many people are genuinely motivated to test their limits, to see how far they can take self-improvement in every realm, including the physical. There is something magical about looking in the mirror and witnessing the changes in the way your body looks, and knowing that you were personally responsible for that change. Creating an increased capacity for physical work is extremely empowering — discovering that you can lift objects heavier than you used to lift, or walk farther and more comfortably than you used to walk.

People who want to engage in physically demanding recreational activities, from hiking to skiing to rock climbing, also benefit from regular fitness training because it reduces the likelihood of injury. Plus, the regimen inherent in fitness training is also a good way to learn the discipline that might be useful in other areas of life. The ability to set goals and follow them through, to manage time, to conserve energy until just the right moment -- these are all useful skills to have. Physical fitness, precisely because of its "material" nature, makes the lesson of discipline easier to appreciate.

Wellness

Sometime in the early 1990's, I began hearing people in the fitness industry use the word "wellness" to indicate that there was more to being in good condition than just physical fitness. They recognized, for example, that there was also a strong psychological component, and the need to reduce disease risk factors like smoking or poor nutrition. But what, exactly, is "wellness?"

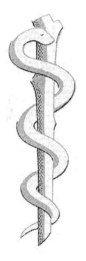

According to Webster's dictionary, "wellness" is the antonym -- the opposite - of illness. If by "illness" we mean to describe a state of being injured or diseased in some way, then the opposite of that is a state in which you are free from overt, acute or chronic conditions of injury or sickness. In other words, "wellness" is based on a medical model, and focuses on the soundness of the bodily functions.

Wellness is not only different from fitness by definition; it is also a condition that *everyone* desires. Even couch potatoes want to be well - they're just not happy about the effort required. Unfortunately for the couch potato, true wellness is "behavioral," which means we achieve and maintain a well state of being through our own lifestyle habits and choices. Learning how to eat right, manage stress and exercise in an appropriate way (appropriate for who you are and what is going on your life) can keep you from becoming ill, and can often make the illnesses you have disappear without the use of drugs or surgery.

Dr. Dean Ornish's "healthy heart program" is a good example of how new lifestyle habits bring about wellness. Dr. Ornish is a cardiologist and researcher at the University of California who created a program for reversing heart disease. Heart attacks and atherosclerosis (clogging of the arteries) are the number one causes of death in this country. The common wisdom before Ornish's new program was that heart disease could not be reversed without the use of drug therapy. Moreover, according to Conventional theory, the kinds of exercise required to produce healthy physical benefits for the heart were necessarily aerobic workouts to increase the heart capacity. But Dr. Ornish's program consists entirely of lifestyle changes including a strict vegetarian diet, stress management techniques and group therapy, and exercise that is relaxing rather than stimulating, specifically yoga and walking.

There are two significant and unique aspects of Dr. Ornish's program. First of all, it is entirely drug-free. The entire program is based on activating the wellness systems within a person's own body and mind. And secondly, Dr. Ornish's research data seem to indicate that the program works precisely because the people in the program were active participants in their own wellness program. The more a patient adheres to the lifestyle changes of diet, stress management and exercise, the greater the favorable changes in their condition.

What's the Difference?

Why is it so important to understand the difference between fitness and wellness? Well, suppose you work in a hospital or clinic where you offer exercise for "wellness." The effects of your exercise classes should be to develop the habits that prevent future disease or injury. A "fitness" class -- a class designed to improve athletic performance -- is out of place here. A T'ai Chi class, a restorative yoga class, a walking program, or a Pilates-type conditioning class: these would be appropriate. A step-aerobics class, or a bodybuilding type weight-training workout: these would not be appropriate.

You might ask, "doesn't wellness imply a higher degree of fitness?" Well, yes... usually wellness does accompany improvement in all the components of fitness (strength, flexibility, agility, balance, endurance). But a fitness workout is by definition designed to focus on *optimizing performance or appearance,* while a wellness workout by definition is designed to *restore functionality and ingrain positive lifestyle habits.*

The point I'm trying to make is that people exercise for different reasons, for different purposes, different desired effects and feelings. When exercise authorities offer identical workouts regardless of the environment, they have failed to honor the diversity of needs among people. And this is particularly significant because most exercise professionals are trained to teach "fitness" workouts, but only a minority of people is really interested in greater fitness.

The lack of semantic clarity confuses both the people who are trying to promote wellness and the people who are trying to *find* wellness. When the average person finds a program that advertises wellness but which has an exercise component that actually promotes fitness, their activity ultimately detracts from the exercise experience. Not only does it detract from the experience, but also it literally takes up space that could be filled with a wellness promoting activity.

Several years ago I began a T'ai Chi program for the cardiac rehab center at Queen's Hospital in Honolulu. When I walked into the lab on my first visit, I found it was filled with treadmills and exercise cycles. While I recognize that these tools are practical approaches to getting people to move their bodies, their presence in the lab had become a tacit message that most of the patients had unconsciously interpreted as *the way* to make themselves well again. Many of them had made that decision because when they walked into the cardiac rehab center these were the exercise tools that were there.

The men and women in the cardiac rehab program didn't realize that the treadmills, bicycles and weight machines that filled their lab space were actually designed to promote *fitness*, rather than wellness or health. Their time and energy were being spent on activities designed to make them just look better, convinced that the treadmills and weight machines would fix what was wrong with them.

Health

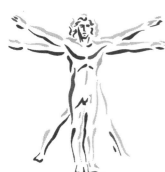

Finally, there is a state of being that incorporates both fitness and wellness, but also exceeds them. This is the state known as "health," a word whose roots go back to the old English word "hale" which means *whole*. Health is a state of wholeness -- and focuses not just on the body, but on the mind and spirit as well. Whereas fitness is based on an athletic model, and wellness is based on a medical model, health is based on a spiritual model.

If our exercise practices are always focused on "optimizing results," we need to be aware that taken to its extreme, exercising may actually be bad for you -- may actually make you "ill" rather than well, or disconnected and un-whole rather than healthy. In my practice as a teacher of mind/body exercise, I have met literally hundreds of people who have exercised themselves into injury and stress. For example, studies have shown that women who furiously involve themselves in intense aerobic exercise on a regular basis may develop Epstein-Barr syndrome, and go through years of the cycle of depression. Here's another example: one of my students was a professional dancer/athlete who worked out for years on a painful foot. When he finally went to the doctor, he was told, "You've been dancing on a stress fracture for years, and now it's so bad that now I'm going to recommend that you can't exercise at all."

To be whole is to have the body, mind and spirit present, associated, and integrated with each other - not separated out, repressed or denied in some way. And when body, mind and spirit come together, a magical thing happens. In that moment of the runners' high, the tennis players' zone, or the yogi's samadhi, there is peace, wholeness, a quality of life that we call, "soul."

The search for health can also be called a search for wholeness, a search for *soulfulness*. The opposite of being whole is being compartmentalized, to cut pieces out of ourselves away from each other. In other words, what brings you wholeness is perhaps an activity that is different from the activities of fitness or wellness, which tend to focus on *parts* of the body. So if you want to be whole you logically need to do something that trains you to be integrated rather than compartmentalized.

As long as exercise feels like work instead of play, most people will never make it a priority. How do we make exercise as much a part of our day as eating and sleeping? We have to make it feel connected to the rest of life. The mind/body approach is a way of making working out a more Holistic event. Soulful exercise is always a multidimensional experience, not a singular "task" Soulful exercise is exercise with the entire being turned "on," with the mind and spirit alert and ready to experience the soul because of the way that the body interacts with the environment, and with itself. In the next chapter, we'll begin to explore what happens if we change the basic paradigm that guides the way we think about exercise in this culture. The first step is to acknowledge that in addition to being inherently perfect and complete, we are also each uniquely different and diverse. Perhaps, if we learn how to move with soul, then we can also understand how soul moves us.

Desideratum #2: The Three Continua

Very soon we will begin to construct a program for your life, and you will need the three continua to select your elements. This mini-chapter is also a gift. Open it, and I hope to hear you say, "I can now see a way of creating order out of the seeming-chaos of all the possible choices in exercise, stress management and diet."

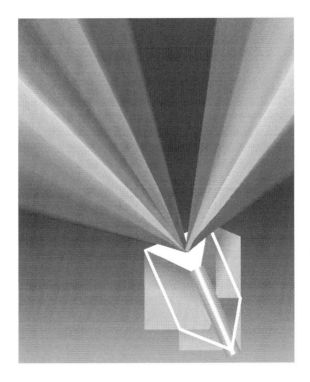

Three Continua (Exercise, Diet, Relaxation)

The Workout Continuum was one of the first tools I developed to help my students and clients choose the right kind of exercise. I started by noticing that there was a very real difference between the experience of lifting weights or doing other mainstream types of exercise, and the experience of practicing yoga or T'ai Chi Ch'uan. This led me to dividing workouts into two types – Conventional and Mind/Body. Later, as I distinguished that there was also a difference between the ancient disciplines like T'ai Chi and the more modern formats like Pilates, I made a middle-of-the-road category. Finally I realized that what I was seeing was a spectrum – a gradual transition between the two extremes of design: reductive and integrative. Whether they knew it or not, the inventors of different workouts were crafting their exercises somewhere along that spectrum. The workout continuum is a model to shows approximately where a particular movement activity lies along that design spectrum.

That's all very interesting, you may say, but how does this help *me*? Well, after we've assessed our wellness lifestyle practices through the Wellness Index, the next logical question is something like, "OK, so now what do I *do?*" How does one choose the "right" workout, diet or stress management technique?

The Holistic approach suggests that the way to make choices is to consider first the BodyMind type of the individual, and the universal compensations and/or core dynamics at work. We then try to align the masks we've discovered with the activity or regimen appropriate to the BodyMind season. And we assess what is "appropriate" by understanding the design of each available choice, and the likely effect of that design.

Design 101

As we create and design a thing, we include a variety of specific elements in its design, so that it will eventually perform a particular function or functions. You make a thing so that it will do something particular for you. For example, if you want a vehicle to propel you down the highway, you design a comfortable carriage, put four wheels on it, and give it an engine, drive shaft and differential. But more specific design elements will make your vehicle unique, and different from other cars. For example, if you want your vehicle to be environmentally friendly, you substitute an electric motor for the gas-burning engine. The design elements, therefore, give it a particular character, and the character reflects the paradigm in which it was created.

Every workout, diet or relaxation technique "works," and is therefore appropriate for somebody, somewhere, at some time. One isn't faced with an either/or choice. Instead, we can understand that our lifestyle options are sprinkled like rainbow colors across spectra that connect polar opposites of design features. Workouts, for example, fall along a continuum that is less integrative on one end, and very integrative on the other end. Diets range from those that are food oriented to those that are "people-oriented;" and relaxation methods are arrayed from those that are externally generated to those that are generated from within.

The Workout Continuum

(simplified)

- Muscular Strength
- Endurance
- Flexibility
- Cardio-pulmonary
- Body Composition

- Integration
- Therapeutic Rebalancing
- Emotional Freedom

- Alignment
- Visualization
- Breath Control
- Relaxation
- ***Inner Energy***

⇐ Conventional   Modern Mind/Body   Classical Mind/Body ⇒

Less Integrative   *More Integrative*

- Weight Training
- Aerobics
- Sports Conditioning
- Spinning
- Body Pump

- Pilates
- Nia
- Flow Motion
- Feldenkrais
- Systematic T.O.U.C.H.
- ***Something New***

- Hatha Yoga
- Pranayama
- T'ai Chi Ch'uan
- Ch'i Kung

Conventional Exercise

At the far left end of the continuum, where the Conventional paradigm is at home, we find workouts that are designed in the Conventional way, like weight training and the various aerobic and conditioning classes, and which focus on developing very physical and mechanical attributes. For example, weight lifting builds muscular strength, which is necessary for lifting, jumping, pulling and punching. Aerobic exercise, like aerobic dance classes, running, swimming and bicycling, builds endurance and increases the capacity of the heart and lungs.

Modern Mind/Body Exercise

As we progress along the spectrum towards greater integration, workouts begin to *transcend* the physical aspects of exercise, although they certainly include them. In other words, workout designs begin to grow towards greater integration, not only of body, but also of mind and Spirit. We call these the "modern" mind/body exercises. They focus on bringing the mind and the body together, not only working out the body, but also teaching you how to be aware of every part of the body as it is working – even down to the cellular and energetic level. Modern mind/body workouts also teach you how to exercise in a way that reduces stress and conserves your life force so that you can enjoy the feeling of health and vitality during an extraordinarily long life.

One could say that Modern mind/body exercise strengthens your ability to "think" with your body and "move" with your mind. Physical exercise may make your muscles bigger, but only mind/body exercise can enable you to be aware of disease or injury days before any symptoms show themselves. These are fairly recent experiments (within the last 100 years) in integrating the body, mind and spirit, like Nia (Neuromuscular Integrative Action) and Pilates-inspired workouts, which are characterized by a vocabulary full of words like "feeling," "observing" and integrating.

Classical Mind/Body Exercise

At the far right end of the spectrum, finally, we find the "classical" mind/body workouts. Classical mind/body workouts, which include hatha yoga, pranayama, T'ai Chi Ch'uan and ch'i kung. According to the traditions of these arts, the body, mind and Spirit are already integrated. What is sometimes missing is a sense of these parts operating together synergistically; therefore these workouts are actually designed to develop synergy. They are also designed to awaken the life energy within the individual. These are the workouts that focus on the development, conservation and circulation of vital life energy (i.e. ch'i, ki and prana). Furthermore, all of them are characterized by the careful attention to alignment of the spine, use of breath in concert with movement, movement done with relaxation, and the use of visualization.

Every one of these exercises utilizes mind/body integration as a *means* to positively affect vital energy flow. The healthier and more balanced the flow of your energy, the healthier you are. Moreover, every one of these disciplines maintains that only movement *done in a certain way* will have this positive effect. The teachings of ch'i kung, T'ai Chi and yoga are specific: movements must be done in a state of relaxation, in concert with the breath, with mind-directed movement of energy, and with the spine in a specific alignment.

Of course, as we look more closely at some of the workouts within each category, we start to find that many workouts seem to cross over the lines. For example, Systematic T.O.U.CH. Training is a Conventional workout -- a weight lifting method -- that emphasizes more of the cognitive and affective aspects, like a true mind/body workout. Likewise, Flow Motion is a modern mind/body workout, but is designed to adhere to the characteristics of classical mind/body disciplines, such as emphasizing posture, breath and visualization.

If, as I have said, we take a step towards wholeness when we integrate ourselves and we take step away from wholeness when we compartmentalize ourselves, then we take a step away from health the closer we are to the less integrative end of the spectrum and we take a step towards health when we choose workouts from the more integrative end. Conventional workouts by design are less integrative and therefore less concerned with health. Mind/body workouts – particularly classical mind/body workouts – by design are more integrative and therefore more concerned with health.

The Diet Continuum

Much like the workout continuum, the diet continuum is a way to look at all the possible diets in the world, laid out in a way that makes it easier to make choices for your own program.

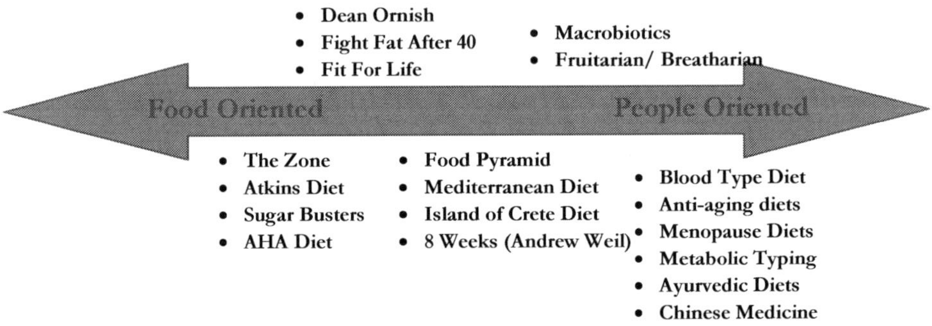

Food Oriented ←——————————————→ **People Oriented**

Above the axis:
- Dean Ornish
- Fight Fat After 40
- Fit For Life
- Macrobiotics
- Fruitarian/ Breatharian

Below the axis:
- The Zone
- Atkins Diet
- Sugar Busters
- AHA Diet

- Food Pyramid
- Mediterranean Diet
- Island of Crete Diet
- 8 Weeks (Andrew Weil)

- Blood Type Diet
- Anti-aging diets
- Menopause Diets
- Metabolic Typing
- Ayurvedic Diets
- Chinese Medicine

Define "diet." If you said, "a way to lose weight," then you might be missing a more basic definition of the word – which is simply "what do you eat?" Let's use the word to *de*scribe rather than *pre*scribe the way you make nutritional choices.

People make up diets, just like they make up exercise routines. Diets reflect all sorts of ideas and influences, like ethnic culture or special medical needs. But one way of looking at how diets are designed is whether they are "people-oriented" or "food-oriented."

Food-oriented diets center around the food itself in the diet. The most extreme expression of this orientation is purely the chemical nature of the food. What is the nutritional and/or caloric value of the food you're eating? Barry Sears' Zone Diet and the Atkins Diet are two examples of food-oriented diets.

People-oriented diets, on the other hand, revolve around the people who are eating the food. These diets consider that the same food might actually affect two different people in very different ways. Pasta, bread or rice, for example, might be the perfect staple for certain individuals whereas for others it causes nothing but bloating, indigestion or weight-gain.

The question is, from which end of the continuum should you be eating? Well, obviously there is no single right or wrong way to eat. Each individual discovers the foods that nourish or weaken. And just like physical workouts, statistics show that almost every diet "works" – if you stick to them. The single factor that seems to predict whether someone will be successful in their dietary goals is how long they actually stick to the diet.

Again, just like physical workouts, your diet has both a physical impact as well as an emotional one. Supposing you are an Indian Summer – a communi-verted individual, motivated by human relationships. If you try to eat according to diets from the left end of the diet continuum – the food-oriented diets – you are likely to have an emotionally difficult time sticking to it. These diets, although they may be chemically accurate and technically impeccable, leave the temperament of the people involved out of the equation, and you are a "people person." On the other hand, if you try to eat according to diets from the right side of the continuum – the people-oriented diets – you are likely to have an emotionally easy time sticking to it.

The Relaxation Continuum

Much like the workout continuum, the Relaxation continuum is a way to look at all the possible stress management techniques in the world, laid out in a way that makes it easier to make choices for your own program.

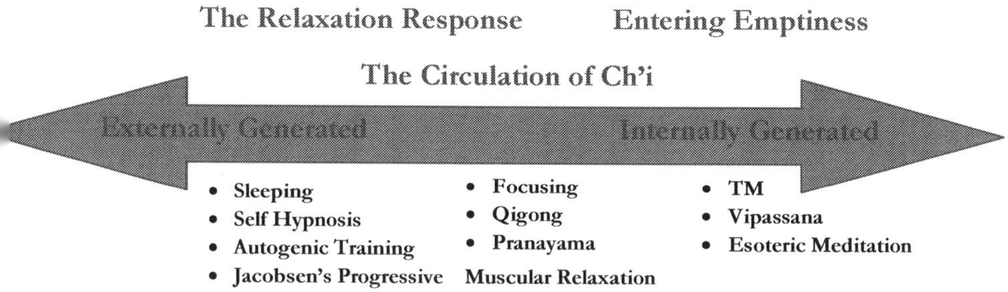

The Relaxation Response — Entering Emptiness

The Circulation of Ch'i

Externally Generated ← → **Internally Generated**

- Sleeping
- Self Hypnosis
- Autogenic Training
- Jacobsen's Progressive Muscular Relaxation

- Focusing
- Qigong
- Pranayama

- TM
- Vipassana
- Esoteric Meditation

What is stress? There are many different ways of defining stress, beginning with the definition written by Hans Selye, the man often called the Father of modern stress theory. One way we can define stress in a measurable way is to say that stress is the over activation of the sympathetic nervous system and the renal cortex.

Therefore, the opposite of that stress is to sedate the sympathetic nervous system – which is what happens when you activate the parasympathetic nervous system. What do we call activating the parasympathetic? We call it relaxation. Dr. Herb Benson from the Harvard Medical School has written a book and done considerable research on something he calls, "the relaxation response."

Think of stress management as the ability to stay relatively relaxed in the face of stressors, or to bring you back to balance when you encounter stressors. One way of gauging whether or not you are out of balance is to ask if you are being productive. The Yerkes-Dodson Law says that stress will improve performance up to a certain point, after which performance will worsen. If you're chronically over-stressed, then it doesn't take much to push you over the "edge" into decreased performance.

Stress management can be seen as "relaxing" in the face of inner and/or outer conflict or inner and/or outer relationships. The question is: what method do *you* use to relax? Like physical activity and diet, one technique does not fit all people. A variety of different techniques, however, will create the variety of choices that open the experience of balance for more people. There may be many different ways of describing the design elements of all the stress management techniques, but one I've used for years is to consider that these techniques can be either "internally generated" or "externally generated."

As I use these terms, internal means coming from inner thoughts or emotions. The most extreme examples of internally generated relaxation techniques are the esoteric meditations taught by many spiritual traditions. On the other end of the continuum are relaxation techniques that start with the body. These are the externally generated methods. The relaxation here works from the outside in, as opposed to the inside out.

Like both the workout continuum and the diet continuum, the way to use the relaxation continuum is to consider whom you are and why you want to relax. For instance, if you are one of the BodyMind types whose temperament is typically less spiritual or intuitive, then you might have an easier time using one of the techniques that starts from the outside, focusing on the body and its sensations. On the other hand, if you might be one of the Seasons who are introspective and Spiritual by temperament. You might have an easier time using one of the techniques that starts from the inside, focusing the mind and pursuing the state of samadhi, or enlightenment.

Chapter IV: Kinesiology

There is a skill to interpreting what you see in the mirror or observe how you move through space. The gift of the fourth chapter, Kinesiology, is *skill*. In this chapter you will learn to look at yourself in the mirror in an informed and enlightened way. You'll start to learn to. Open this gift, and I hope to hear you say, "I begin to see the patterns molded into my body – both literally and figuratively."

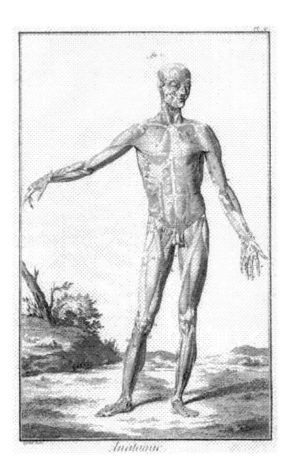

The Science of Motion

The human body, at its most basic level of organization is made up of cells. Cells combine to make tissue, and specialized groups of tissue make up our organs, muscles and bones. Every cell is like a little factory. It takes in the raw materials of nutrients and oxygen it gets from the blood, combines them with its own internal chemicals and creates a "product" – the unique function it was made to perform. The by-products of a cell's work are waste gases and toxins, disposed of at last through the excretory system.

Motion inspires the lively operation of each cell in many ways. For example, movement stimulates the lungs to open up to larger volumes of air, to gather oxygen into the bloodstream. That same movement causes the heart to pump blood into the circulatory system, carrying that oxygen, along with life-giving nutrients from our digested food, in each little cell. On its way out of the cell, that same blood, pumped by that same heart, stimulated by the same movement, carries the metabolic wastes and toxins out of the cell to be disposed of.

The study of how the human body moves is called "kinesiology." At rest, the human body stands ready to move in what is known as an anatomically neutral position, held in place by a synergy of muscles on all sides that keep the bones stable. We basically move through space because body parts bend and reach. Our bones articulate at the joints, because a well-coordinated group of muscles exert a pull on one end of a bone, like the chain attached to the lip of a drawbridge. As the muscles exert more pull, the bones move more. The muscles themselves exert their pull because nerves fire at the ends of the muscle fibers, causing them to contract. And the whole process of movement begins when a thought – whether conscious, unconscious or reactive – sends a message to the nerves to commence firing.

Part of the science of kinesiology is to consider what happens when something throws the delicate coordination of thoughts, nerves, muscles and bones out of balance. Imagine the pelvis, held in place by a company of stabilizing muscles throughout the lower back, pelvic floor, gluteal and abdominal areas, connected to both the spine and the legs. What would happen if one of those stabilizing muscles started to exert too much pull, as muscles do when they spasm? Slowly the pelvis would be pulled toward the overactive muscle, shifting it out of its neutral alignment. The other stabilizers would have to unnaturally lengthen to accommodate the new position of the bone. The gait pattern would be altered, as now the shifted pelvis affected the operation of the legs. And most likely there would be pain, as now the bones, muscles and connective tissue were dragged into new positions where they unwillingly pressed on the nerves.

When we are sedentary, the operations of each little factory begin to grind to a halt. The waste management system slows down, and toxins begin to accumulate in our cells, sometimes to the point of killing the cell itself. Aging is a phenomenon of the body's decreasing ability over time to keep the body's cells healthy and alive. When our inner systems no longer support our ability to move, our bodies think that we're ready to die.

When my father was in the hospital after being diagnosed with cancer, I started to teach him Tai Chi Ch'uan. Nothing fancy, just shifting the weight slowly forward and back. We stood in the hospital hallway, and I showed him how to withdraw his hands into his chest when he went back, circle them down, then up, and then push his palms our when he rocked forward. I told him to imagine running his thumbs around a dinosaur egg. In the middle of this, Dad's oncologist walked by and asked what we were doing. "I'm teaching Dad to do T'ai Chi," I said. The doctor watched us for minute. "I wish I could get all my patients to do this," he said. I watched him walk away, shaking his head, and I wondered if he was thinking what I was thinking: that I wished I had taught my father T'ai Chi *before* he learned he had cancer.

The systems of the human body – its organs, fluids, nerves, bones and muscles – are designed to adapt to environmental demands. The natural life of every cell depends upon the stimulus of a certain amount of physical movement. Your body *assumes* you are going to make it work. The heart and lungs, for example, want a reason to pump blood and gulp oxygen out of the air. Without movement, the metabolism slows down, toxins accumulate and our brains "forget" how to coordinate the firing of nerves and the flexing of muscles. We atrophy. We age. We begin to die.

At the same time, there is a Spirit within the body that wants to live. When we slow down because of age, illness, injury or stress, the body begins to try to compensate for the change. These compensations, as I have said before, are the body's attempt to restore functionality. They are at the same time messages to the conscious mind, inviting it engage in a conversation. "Pay attention to me," the body is saying. "I'm out of balance."

A Body Out of Balance

Trauma of any kind upsets the balance of your body. Obviously, physical trauma impacts our muscles, nerves and bones – but so does mental or emotional trauma. And when we have a physical trauma, which could be anything from a train wreck to the flu to getting out of shape and gaining weight, it has an unbalancing effect on our thoughts, emotions and Spirit.

On a structural level, we call imbalances "postural distortions." In Tables 1, 2 and 3, you will find some of the most common postural distortions to be found in the human body. When you read the tables, you'll probably notice that some of the distortions are familiar – they're in your own body! Notice that in line with a particular symptom are two columns -- one for muscles that are overly tight *and* a column for muscles that are weak and loose. This is because in the human body, muscles are typically paired around the bones and joints. In their ideal synergy, the muscle pairs exert forces to appropriately accelerate, decelerate or stabilize the body parts. But when a trauma occurs, suddenly there is an imbalance in the ability of one or both of the muscle pair to do its job. When one of the pair tightens up, or gets shorter, it pulls on the other one, lengthening and loosening it. Now neither one can create a strong contraction.

Compensations and Muscle Imbalances

Postural Distortions	Tight Muscles	Weak Muscles
Foot and Ankle Complex		
Feet Flatten	Gastrocnemius, Peroneals	Gluteus Medius, Anterior Tibialis, Posterior Tibialis
Feet Externally Rotate	Soleus, Biceps Femoris, Piriformis	Gluteus Medius
Knees		
Knees Adduct	Adductors, Iliotibial band	Gluteus Medius, Gluteus Maximus
Knees Abduct	Biceps femoris, Iliopsoas, Piriformis	Gluteus Medius, Gluteus Maximus

Table 1

Table 2

Lumbo-Pelvic-Hip Complex		
Asymmetrical Weight Shifting	Gastrocnemius, Soleus, Biceps Femoris, Adductors, Iliotibial Band, Iliopsoas, Piriformis	Gluteus Medius, Gluteus maximus, Transversus Abdominus, Multifidi
Increased Lumbar Extension	Iliopsoas, Rectus Femoris, Erector Spinae, Latissimus Dorsi	Gluteus Maximus/Medius, Lumbo-Pelvic-Hip complex stabilization mechanism
Increased Lumbar Flexion	External Obliques, Rectus Abdominus, Hamstrings	Gluteus Maximus/Medius, Lumbo-Pelvic-Hip complex stabilization mechanism
Abdomen Protrudes	Iliopsoas	Lumbo-Pelvic-Hip complex stabilization mechanism

Shoulder Complex		
Arms Fall Forward (when overhead) or Lumbar Spine Hyperextends	Latissimus dorsi, Pectoralis Major	Middle/Lower Trapezius
Elbows Flex (when arms are overhead)	Pectoralis Major	Middle/Lower Trapezius
Shoulder Blade Abducted	Upper Trapezuis, Levator Scapulae, Pectoralis Major/Minor	Rhomboids, Middle/Lower Trapezius
Shoulder Blade Protracted	Pectoralis Major/Minor, Latissimus Dosi	Rhomboids, Middle/Lower Trapezius, Teres Minor, Infraspinatus
Shoulder Elevated	Upper Trapezius, Levator Scapulae	Lower Trapezius
Shoulder Blade Winging	Pectoralis Minor	Serratus Anterior, Lower Trapezius

Table 3

Exercise

The mysteriograph is an optical illusion – a painting that looks like nothing more than meaningless dots and swirls. But if you look at it long enough, slightly crossing your eyes and unfocusing your gaze, a new picture emerges, previously hidden in the dots and swirls. Looking in the mirror, what do you see? The same old face and body you saw yesterday. Yet if you were to look at yourself in a different way, you might see a new image emerge, hidden in the familiarity of your own reflection.

Start by separating your body into parts: lower, middle and upper. The lower body section includes the feet, ankles, knees and legs. The middle body section, which is technically referred to as the "lumbo-pelvic-hip complex," includes the hips, waist and lower back. Finally, the upper body section includes the torso, arms, hands, elbows, shoulders and head.

For now, just try to notice what your body looks like at seven different specific locations feet, ankles, knees, hips, waist, shoulders and head. In particular, look for differences from one side of the body to the other, and compare your reflection with the postural distortions noted on Tables 1-3.

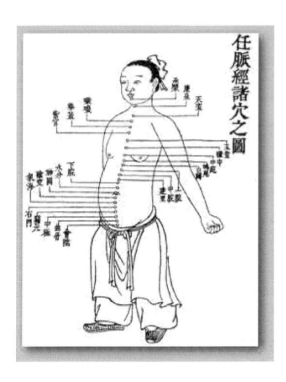

Head

Shoulders
 (back)

Hips (waist)

Knees

Feet (ankles)

What do you see?

Feet: _____

_____

Knees: _____

_____

Hips: _____

_____

Torso: _____

_____

Shoulders: _____

_____

Head: _____

_____

A Glossary of Symptoms

- Monoplanar movement
    - The tendency to move in the same plane or planes (i.e. saggital, frontal or transverse).
- Extreme linearity
    - The tendency to move (and even think) in straight lines.
- Over-activity
    - Muscles that don't relax but are perpetually contracting.
- Hypertonicity
    - Another version of overactivity, where the muscles are in a constant state of contraction, appearing extremely "toned," and in a state of flexion all the time.
- Muscle imbalance
    - Muscles usually appear in the body in pairs – like biceps or deltoids on the right and left side of the body. For a variety of reasons, muscles may develop more on one side. Also, over-stressed or injured muscles may spasm, creating a condition in which one set of muscles are in a constant state of over-activity, or even shut off and become atrophied.
- Chronic overuse injury
    - Over-stressing a muscle leads to injury, often times in the connective tissue. This comes from repeated use of the muscle in the same pattern of motion – usually a compensatory pattern.
- Dissociation
    - This is the term we give to complete disconnection from (and in some sense, rejection of) our bodies.
- Atrophy
    - Remember the phrase, "Use it or lose it?" That principle is very true when it comes to your body's strength and function. When muscles are unused for a long period of time, they begin to shrink and weaken, literally withering away while the nerves go to sleep.

- Severe debilitating injury
    - Accidents and injuries can occur in many different places – the home, the workplace, even in sports and recreational settings. Sometimes these injuries can be so severe that they cause the body to shut down in some areas for a long period of time.
- Underactivation
    - Sometimes muscles can be slow to fire that they seem to be asleep. In fact, they are often not getting a strong signal from the nerves that activate them. This sometimes occurs from being underused, or from an injury. After a time, even when a signal comes from the brain to activate that muscle, the resulting contraction is either slow to occur, or weak – or both.
- Lack of proprioception
    - The proprioceptors are a special class of nerves that help sense the body's position in space, its relationship to other objects and how the body is moving. They are located throughout the body in the skin, in the muscles, at the joints – even in the inner ear. When one is not used to being physical, it is common for the brain to have a hard time interpreting the signals the proprioceptors are sending. Proprioceptors sometimes turn off and don't function as accurate sensors. In either case, we call this a "lack of proprioception," signaling a lowered kinesthetic "sense-ability."
- Inactive core
    - The muscles of the thoracic core – the abdominals, the lower back, the pelvic floor and glutes – are the essential muscles of stabilization in the body. Metaphorically, these muscles are the center of your physical being. A common phenomenon I see among both men and women are weak or completely inactive core muscles.
- Altered force couple (postural distortion)
    - Every bone or body segment is connected to a pair (or group) of muscles that in tandem both move and stabilize that body part. Each muscle individually exerts a force on the bone, and the balance of all the forces is called a "force couple." When one muscle goes weak and slack – or goes into spasm and pulls too much – the force couple is altered. The altered force couple is an imbalance, and begins to pull the body part out of alignment, creating a postural distortion.

- Synergistic dominance
    - Big muscles, with the help of some other smaller muscles that guide, stabilize and support it, move most of our body parts. The big muscles are called "prime movers," and the helper muscles are called "synergists." When the big muscles stop working efficiently – as after an injury, or a resulting pattern of compensation – the synergist take over to take up the slack. After a time, the body gets used to the synergists causing the motion of body parts that used to by the responsibility of the prime movers. Now the body habitually by-passes the activation of the prime movers, and the synergists do the work instead. This is called "synergistic dominance."
- Weight shifting
    - As the body moves through space – back and forth, side to side, turning, or up and down – the body should evenly transfer weight from one foot to the other. If, however, you see yourself habitually shifting one foot, favoring the other side, we call this an abnormal weight shift.
- Inflexibility and Pain
    - Although we might not think of these as postural distortions, inflexibility and pain can limit the way we move – the way we experience our bodies. Pain and inflexibility can show up as patterns in our bodies that diminish the experience of power, freedom and flow.

A Final Thought

If you were to look in the mirror, could you pick out your own compensations and postural distortions? Don't worry – it gets easier with practice. What you'll see first are the most obvious *symptoms,* and then patterns and combinations of these symptoms. Very soon you will be able to distinguish on your own which of the 6 Universal Compensations are at work in your own body.

By following these compensations to their source, you will finally discover the deep and fundamental dynamic at work – in fact one of the three core dynamics. Only by distinguishing these dynamics – these primary masks – will you be able to travel very far on your journey to health.

The thing to recognize about our patterns, compensations and masks is that while we build them from the inside out, we discover them from the outside in. In the Conventional paradigm, the pattern of your tapestry is interpreted as physical dysfunctions that need to be fixed or improved to achieve optimal performance. There is another way to look in this mirror, however. Instead of literally analyzing the muscles, nerves and bones of your body, imagine that your body is made up of a series of conversations. In the Holistic paradigm, these so-called physical dysfunctions are the body's way of talking to you, asking you to take notice of a pattern of behavior that is masking wholeness.

What do you do if you can't figure out what your body is showing you?

1. Look to the next level – the patterns themselves – and see if the descriptions of the patterns resonate with you in any way.
2. Remember, more than one pattern can be present simultaneously. What we're looking for is the strongest or most dominant pattern. This is another version of the weakest link.
3. Don't forget my invitation to use the website, www.thewellnessevolution.com, to look up references and view case studies. If possible, send us a digital photo, and we'll work with you to complete your assessment, and help you hone your skills.

A word of caution: Do not get overly caught up in the physical body, since your body is also a mirror for the rest of your life. The body is merely the most material aspect of ourselves, and therefore the easiest to see, touch, feel and measure. But the symptoms, patterns and masks you discover in your body are also occurring in your way of thinking and feeling. In other words, as we use the lens of kinesiology to distinguish our patterns and then implement a workout, a diet or a technique for calming ourselves, remember that although your actions may feel body-centered, they will also be creating ripples of change in your psyche and Spirit.

Chapter V: Conversations of the Body

The gift of the fifth chapter, Conversations of the Body, is *insight*. It's so easy sometimes to throw up our hands and say, "Something is wrong with me!" Open this gift, however, and I hope to hear you say, "I see myself as I never have before. I see there is nothing to fix, only masks to undo."

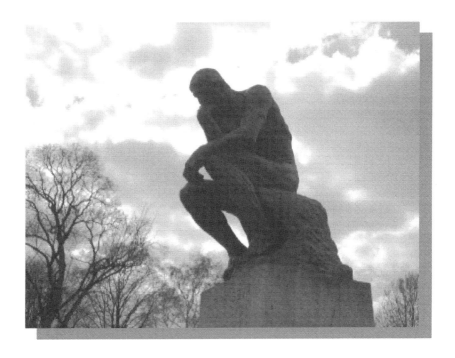

The Body as Metaphor

Even some of my closest friends and loyal students sometimes have a hard time holding onto the philosophy of "there's nothing wrong – you're perfect." When your body is in pain, when you begin to feel the weight of your years, or when you look into the mirror and see a pear where you hoped to see an hourglass, the most natural thing in the world is to say to ourselves that something *is* terribly, terribly wrong.

But what if everything you felt in your body, or saw when you looked in the mirror wasn't taken literally? What if you could see that every pain and every pattern of compensation is actually an invitation to a conversation that your body wants to have with your mind. Your discomforts are a call to a journey within to find your authentic self.

The mystical traditions of many cultures share a concept that can be expressed, "As above, so below." In the T'ai Chi Classics, the ancient Masters say, "The inner matches the outer." In other words, the body is a metaphor for the rest of your life, and whatever is manifesting on the physical level (pain, imbalance, weakness, tension, tightness, looseness, etc.) is present on the emotional, mental and Spiritual levels as well.

> *"The primary markers of physical capacity are strength, endurance, flexibility and resilience. These are precisely the same markers of capacity emotionally, mentally, and spiritually. Mental endurance is a measure of the ability to sustain focus and concentration over time, while mental flexibility is marked by the capacity to move between the rational and the intuitive and to embrace multiple points of view. Spiritual strength is reflected in the commitment to one's deepest values, regardless of circumstance and even when adhering to them involves personal sacrifice."* -- The Dynamics of Full Engagement

The body is a metaphor for every area of your life, and whatever is manifesting on the physical level (pain, imbalance, weakness, tension, tightness, looseness, etc.) is surely present on the emotion, mental and Spiritual levels as well.

The conditions, complaints and anxieties of the body are messages, and admittedly most of the time we don't know what those messages mean. But then again, maybe we don't need to know. What is more important is the practice of listening to those messages. If we develop the habit of looking at physical structures and thinking of them metaphorically rather than literally, we may actually begin to see patterns emerge, like looking at the mysteriograph. If you think those illustrations are only a confusing collection of dots and whirls, that's all you'll ever see. But if you know that another picture is hidden inside, and all you have to do is look at it long enough and sooner or later it will leap out at you, in 3-D.

> "Emotions that we cannot allow into consciousness often express themselves somatically, through our body." -- Joan Borysenko

John came to me to find some relief from more than two years of constant pain in his left leg, groin and lower back. He happened to run into one of my students, who recommended T'ai Chi.

John had chased the cause of his pain and symptoms for two years, visiting many specialists – neurologists, urologists, massage therapists, acupuncturists – all without success. No one could find the cause of his condition. When asked to place his pain on a scale of 1-10, he said he had lived for most of those two years with a daily pain level of 7, and found it difficult to sleep at night, or sit for long periods of time.

One of the few moments of relief, he said, came when he took hot baths. In those hot baths John would dig his fingers into the muscles of his legs to try to massage away the pain (mostly without success), stretch himself out in the hot water and to try to "figure out" what could possibly be the cause of his pain.

I began with the assumption that John was inherently perfect, and that rather than trying to find a problem to fix, I was going to embark on a journey of helping him "reveal" his own perfection. I suggested that he continue to take his hot baths, but that he leave off massaging and stretching, and especially leave off trying to figure things out. It occurred to me that John's body was trying to talk to him – to communicate *something* and he was doing everything but listen to it.

I suggested that he just sit and relax in the bath and allow images to arise in his mind. If there was any actual question to ask, it was, "What do you want to tell me?" I wanted him just to observe and take note of whatever came up.

At the end of the first week, John came to a session with a really wonderful story. He had done what I suggested, and just let images in his mind. "I saw my two legs fighting each other," he said. "It was like the right leg was white, the good leg, and the left leg (which had all the pain) was black, the bad leg. And the good leg said the bad leg, 'Why can't you be more like me?'"

I thought it was an extraordinary image. Could it be that there were parts of John that were at odds with others parts? What if the "legs" themselves were also metaphors? Legs take us places, as do our thoughts and emotions. I know that in my own life there have been many times that my mind took me in one direction when my intuition wanted me to go in another. How, we might consider, does the intuition then get our attention to talk about that if not through bodily sensations?

By the way, during the week in which John had his image, his pain level dropped to a 2. Did the conversation with his body cause his pain to drop? I don't know. But I do know that it is quite common for pain on any level (physical, mental, emotional or Spiritual) to suddenly disappear when we find an access under our masks and start to lift them off.

By their very nature, masks are often invisible to the wearer. Most of us have lived with our compensations for so long that we think the way we experience life is either all there is, or the best it can be. So how do we know where our compensations lie? The first thing you can do is check in with your physical body.

Start with these basic self-check questions. First, do you experience "Power" in relationship to your body? Remember, power is *vitality* – literally, the experience of the vital life energy flowing through your body, mind and Spirit. Power is the ability to cause an outcome without the use of strength or force. *Exercise: Look in the mirror and say to yourself, "I am calm and powerful. I have plenty of energy." Now pause and listen. What does your inner voice say about the* current *accuracy of this statement?*

Power is what one experiences when integrity is present. If you miss the feeling of power in your body, then your physical integrity is weak and you've developed some form of compensation to get things done. This compensation (whatever it is) feels like it makes you functional, but in fact it is standing in between you and the experience of vitality and power. The good news, as we will see later, is that when you know that your integrity is the issue you also know the direction of the appropriate healing solution.

The next question is, do you experience "Freedom" in relationship to your body? Freedom, remember, is boundless, uninhibited *acceptance*. Freedom is not constrained in any way, neither by memories of the past, nor by circumstances of the present, nor even by projections of the future. *Exercise: Look in the mirror and say to yourself, "My body moves freely." Now pause and listen. What does your inner voice say about the* current *accuracy of this statement?*

Freedom is what one experiences when compassion and acceptance is present. If you miss the feeling of freedom in your body, then on some level you believe that something is wrong. It might be a small belief, like "I don't have rhythm." It might be a big message, like "I'm too fat/thin/tall/bald/shy/smart/white." Many people do feel that these inner beliefs drive them to strive for higher levels of self-improvement, and are therefore a "functional" thought-form. Yet in fact, these beliefs veil the fact that there is nowhere to go, no achievement to make that will make you more perfect – for in fact right now, at this very moment, you are as perfect and complete as anyone could possibly be. Compassion is knowing and believing that you are perfect just the way you are, at every moment of your life.

The final question in this exercise is, do you experience "Flow" in relationship to your body? Flow is the sense of uninterrupted continuity and connectedness. It is what athletes call the sweet spot, or "being in the zone." Flow is not self-conscious, nor is it passive, awkward or aggressive. Exercise: Look in the mirror and say to yourself, "My movements are smooth and sure. I'm in the zone." Now pause and listen. What does your inner voice say about the current accuracy of this statement?

Flow is what you experience when synergy is present – conscious and unconscious interweaving of all the parts and levels that make up a human being. If you miss the feeling of flow in your body, then in some way or on some level of thought you've defined yourself as a collection of parts, rather than as a unified whole. Of course, this type of mask is common in our culture, since our Western medical science is based on a "reductionist" paradigm. It's reasonable in our society to describe our bodies in terms of parts and systems. We even separate the body from the mind and Spirit in most conversations. But this kind of thinking is an artificial discontinuity. To separate any part of ourselves from any other part is to be less than human, and is the source of all our suffering.

One of the most precious gifts of being human is our capacity to experience life as powerful, free and flowing. When human beings start to experience life in this way, they feel totally connected, like *nothing* is missing. In a way, these three experiences are the mirror opposites of how life occurs when we wear the compensations that mask our wholeness.

Much of the work I do with clients – even the clients who come to me with specific complaints about their physical well-being – is done in conversation. I ask a lot of questions, like the three questions above. Specifically, there is a formula I use that you can also use for yourself. This is what I call Discovery, the process of distinguishing what might be concealing an individual's perfection. As I mentioned above, what conceals our perfection can be seen as the degree to which we have stepped away from balance, or the degree to which we've reduced ourselves into parts. Therefore in the discovery conversation – whether with yourself or with another – you should be listening for thoughts, words or tones of voice that indicate disconnection or imbalance.

The Discovery Process

Discovery works like this: You begin by asking questions, looking in the mirror, and taking note of all the things you see. Everything you do – every new movement activity, every glimpse you catch of yourself as you pass by a shiny window – is an opportunity to discover new things about how your body feels as it holds itself in different shapes, moves through space and performs "work."

As you collect more and more discoveries, you will begin to notice patterns. The patterns can be identified and named, which is a form of Holistic assessment. It's an "Aha! So that's how I hold my shoulders. I've developed a pattern of Lightness!" This assessment is an opportunity to find an access to the real, authentic perfect you that lies hidden under the mask. If you find the pattern of Lightness in your body, you can take a step toward balance by practicing activities that train you to "pay attention" and connect you more deeply to your Self. And as you develop greater balance in you life, you will also feel a sense of greater awareness and perception – which will lead you to the beginning again, making discoveries and seeing yourself with an ever more enlightened eye.

The first step in the discovery conversation is to listen and re-state. Even if you're just talking to yourself, to say, "so what I hear you saying is…" assures the other that you are not making assumptions, judgments, or alterations to what was said.

Next, acknowledge what was said, felt, thought or experienced. There is no right or wrong to one's experience. An event may be described accurately or inaccurately, but an experience just is – and everyone has the right to have his or her experiences validated. The final step is to be generous in your response. (As a note, being generous is giving – or giving up – something that you don't have to.) The purpose for being generous is to train yourself in the emotional perspective that "nothing is wrong." Consider that since you have been living in the conversation of our current "physical culture," you have already been unconsciously trained in the opposite perspective – in other words, you are fundamentally damaged and need fixing.

Looking in the Mirror

Another method of asking your body to reveal the masks you wear is to actually look at how your body stands and moves. What would you see if you took a look in the mirror with a practiced eye? As we learned in the previous chapter, you might see a unique physical tapestry, woven by the history of your life's events, portraying a body of various muscular imbalances and weaknesses, relative degrees of flexibility and balance, a lifted shoulder here, an off-kilter hip over there, and feet that turn out severely down on the ground.

In the conventional paradigm, the pattern of your tapestry is interpreted as physical dysfunctions that need to be fixed or improved to achieve optimal performance. There is another way to look in this mirror, however. Instead of literally analyzing the muscles, nerves and bones of your body, imagine that your body is made up of a series of conversations. In the holistic paradigm, these so-called physical dysfunctions are the body's way of talking to you, asking you to take notice of a pattern of behavior that is masking wholeness.

Unmasking the BodyMind

Looking in the mirror, you are most likely to see a variety of compensations and distortions. But unlike the conventional approach to assessment and program design, which starts from the assumption that something needs to be fixed or improved, the holistic mantra is, "There is nothing wrong here." I re-emphasize, what we are really doing is creating a new *relationship* with our BodyMind, the foundation of which is working together to *uncover and experience an already existing perfection of body, mind and Spirit.*

This is a process of distinguishing what seems to be missing – strength, balance, coordination, joy in movement, calm, relatedness, for example. Those aspects of perfect health that seem to be missing are not in fact absent, but merely concealed in some way. This means that the first step to creating strategies for healing is to name the masks that veil these concealed areas!

Case Study: Finding Freedom

Julia was a beautiful 40-year-old single mother. Tall and lithe, she looked like a fashion model -- a classic Summer type. At the time I met her, she was engaged in a stressful divorce. Initially, Julia came to me because of pain she was having in her neck, back, leg and foot. On our very first session, however, we determined that she was also experiencing a disturbing gradual loss of strength and flexibility. Julia had been a top-level athlete when she was younger, and a competitive swimmer.

To most eyes, Julia did not look like she had anything wrong with her. She appeared to have good muscle tone, and excellent posture. She exhibited very little postural distortions (although I later determined that this was because she was holding herself in rigid control). Julia had lately been taking yoga and Pilates classes to keep strong and flexible, but instead of getting better, she had been getting worse. She found herself less able to create some of the yoga poses properly, or hold them for very long. In one example, sitting in a simple cobbler's pose with the soles of her feet together, she could not get her left knee to open to the floor.

One of the first tests I performed with Julia was Overhead Squat Test, which reveals how one's posture changes during vertical transition – in other words standing in one place with the arms reaching up overhead, sitting down and standing up. When Julia performed this test, I could see a series of postural distortions that weren't apparent when she stood naturally. Every time she did a squat, her feet turned out, her ankles and knees collapsed together and she leaned forward slightly, increasing the sway in her back. She would also wobble a little each time, as though she was losing her balance a bit. Finally, I noticed that her range of motion – the actual distance she was able to move up and down – was limited.

Most interesting to me was the fact that Julia began doing each series of squats perfectly, holding her body in rigid alignment. Yet after only a few repetitions the distortions and compensations appeared as her stabilizing muscles fatigued and went weak.

Julia's core dynamic – her fundamental mask – was what Tom Stone's Core Dynamics model calls "looking for yourself where you are not." One of the things I noticed was that when she began talking about what was going on in her life, she would say things like, "I guess I've got to be logical and strong just like [the lawyers], otherwise they'll take it as a sign of weakness." Yet all the while, there was a part of Julia that didn't feel right about this approach. Her intuition was telling her that she wasn't being herself, but she wasn't listening. And the more she didn't listen, the more she disconnected from herself. Her body began locking itself up, which she experienced as declining flexibility and waning muscular strength.

I could see many core dynamics at play in Julia's case. I knew the nature of the *primary* mask because whenever we allowed that there was nothing wrong with Julia, that she was actually a strong and sensitive woman who deserved to be emotional, and was in fact powerful when she allowed herself to be who she was, she began to cry. Compassion and acceptance of herself was hidden from her, because she was looking for herself everywhere except the one place she could be found – on the inside.

At the same time, Julia was also wearing secondary masks. By trying so hard to be someone she wasn't, she was trying to force an outcome. The mask of force is what people wear when they can't access their sense of power. And since power is what one experiences when integrity is present, I could see that Julia was also leaking integrity.

A Final Thought

Charlotte is an elegant, intelligent woman of deep social values and Spiritual conviction. She is gentle and gifted with a wonderful sense of humor. Charlotte is also in constant pain.

A few years ago she was in an automobile accident, and since then her lower back is in a constant state of spasm. Some days she struggles to walk, and some nights she cannot sleep. Like many of the people I meet, she sought me out because she'd tried everything else. I initially suggested T'ai Chi Ch'uan as a gentle method of restoring her mobility and flexibility. But at her first lesson I found that her body couldn't handle more than 15-20 minutes of even the gentlest motion without intense pain and nausea. After that, I switched to a less rigorous routine of ch'i kung exercises, slowly adding more variations over time.

Charlotte and I have worked together now for nearly a year. I look forward to our appointments because I truly love our conversations, and I admire so much her commitment to "getting better." Paradoxically, she seems just fine when she arrives – her pain is under control, her mood is good and posture is normal. But almost immediately as we start to work together her pain increases and her nausea returns.

At the end of one of our sessions recently, Charlotte commented that it almost felt like during the day she could keep the pain at a distance. She had developed her armor and her "defenses" as she called them. But when she came to her session with me, suddenly she was in a psychic space where she was safe to lower her defenses. And that's when the pain came back.

The pain, I knew, was there all the time, just below the surface and held at bay by Charlotte's willpower. But at what cost? Charlotte's willpower was really only pushing a part of herself away, creating a greater distance between parts of her own body, mind and Spirit.

At a previous meeting, we had discussed why she felt so tired all the time. I pointed out that her body had constructed an intricate web of compensations – her armor and defenses – and it took a tremendous amount of energy to keep them in place. No wonder she had very little energy left for joy and creativity – for Charlotte.

I myself sometimes want to weep to see such a wonderful human being in pain and suffering. And yet, I know that there is another way to think about pain, that it is a part of the process of the Holistic approach.

The Holistic approach to health and happiness is not a quick fix – it is a journey. It is a special kind of journey, an ancient and venerable one. It is the journey of the hero or heroine. In the mythology of many cultures, that voyage always begins with some great and wrenching event, a monumental *pain* of the Spirit. But that event is not really an evil disaster. It is a call, an invitation to embark on the journey.

> *"Crisis is one of the major ways that de-mystification takes place. Crisis causes pattern interruption. The habituated way we are behaving isn't working anymore! A new way of behaving must be sought. The new way requires imagination."* -- John Bradshaw

One of the most important recurrent themes in the hero or heroine's journey is the descent into Hell. At some point, one runs out of options. The map ends, and the reasonable way no longer works. The hero or heroine is finally stuck without clues, and must turn to the mysterious to find his or her way. The journey now leads into the Underworld – the world that is underneath, the world that is in the "un-conscious."

The descent into the Underworld is perilous. One must come with a gift to appease the guardian of the passage – sometimes seen as a monster, sometimes as a ferryman. The gift is a material one like gold or a precious heirloom. In other words, to travel into the underworld one must give something up, something material and precious. And what could be more precious and mundane than your reasonableness?

The hero or heroine must also come into the underworld unarmed and unshielded. Naked, in a way. Or as Charlotte immediately put it, "defenseless." Yet when the hero or heroine's intentions are pure, there is a kind of divine grace that protects the inward traveler.

Your health and happiness are inside you all the time. They are the experiences of life as joyous, Spiritual, powerful, free and flowing – and these experiences are available to you at this very moment if you choose to have them.

What stands in the way of experiencing our health and happiness are our masks, the iron doorway to what lies within us, guarded by monsters. Throw open the doorways! Make the journey. Be happy – be healthy! You have nothing to lose but your pain.

Chapter VI: A Recipe for Transformation

The gift of the sixth chapter, A Recipe for Transformation, is *empowerment*. Here you will actually learn to take the actions necessary to 1) choose the ingredients that bring you into balance and that begin to lift off the mask hiding your perfection, and 2) cook up a program for putting a new structure of life in place. Open this gift, and I hope to hear you say, "I now have the utensils, the supplies and the support I need to build a plan that can work for me."

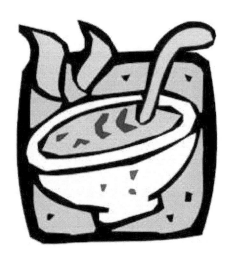

> *"...we must actually do the techniques for them to work. It is a dangerous delusion to substitute knowledge for practice."* -- Ken Pelletier

However more advanced our modern world has become since the days of the wise Chinese doctor and his brother, our lives have now become too sedentary. Our work is in the factory rather than the field, or on the Internet instead of on the ocean; so we need to *add* exercise to keep our bodies fit. Having forgotten to eat the bounty of the earth in the season of its growth, we need to find just the "right" diet. And because we've lost the instinct for rest, play and deep sleep, and because we rarely pay attention to dreams or listen to the village storyteller, we need to plan out and strategically schedule our relaxation.

The practical side of the Holistic approach is to take holistic action. In the Conventional paradigm, fitness trainers refer to their plans for action as, "developing a program." In that culture, the program is written in order to fix or improve something that's wrong with you. An holistic program has a different agenda.

The purpose of every holistic program is to bring your human parts – body, mind, emotions and Spirit – back into balance and connection. As these pieces of you come back together, you will begin to experience more power, freedom and flow in every moment of your life.

The first purpose of your holistic program is to interrupt the cycle of compensations at work in your body – which are the same patterns, by the way, at work in your thoughts and emotions. It is by interrupting these patterns that you begin to peel off the masks that hide your perfection. Since it usually takes more than one time to interrupt/intervene in your pattern, the systematic series of these interruptions is a program.

Even a little crack in the glue that holds your mask in place will invoke the miracle of Spontaneous Healing. Spontaneous Healing is what I call "the magic" that makes the Holistic approach work. The Conventional approach is based on a direct "cause and effect" assumption. Take a pill, and the pill will make your symptoms stop. Lift these weights, and the weight lifting will make your body stronger. But the Holistic approach assumes a different kind of cause and effect relationship. Your perfect body – and mind and Spirit – is always present and just waiting to manifest itself. What it waits for is the clear space to occur. What it waits for is the access, the open doorway into the light of day.

Perhaps this will be clearer if we just look at the body. We heal from illness and injury because the body's immune system goes into action and repairs the hurt, or isolates and "eats up" the disease. Any medications, surgeries or therapies only serve one purpose – to create a condition in which the immune system can do its best work. All the principles and protocols of the Holistic approach combined really only serve one purpose – to create the environment for your own healing to take place. Or said another way, the Holistic approach opens the doorway so that your perfect Self is revealed in the light of day.

The second purpose of every holistic program is to develop new patterns of behavior to take the place of the old ones – patterns that serve to *reveal* your perfection rather than conceal it. Without new ways of moving, thinking or feeling, the old ways will eventually find their way back. Your body, mind, emotions and Spirit will always unconsciously – and automatically – follow the pattern that is most trained. Those patterns have the deepest grooves in our lives. So developing new patterns – patterns that lead back to balance – is also a program.

Finally, the purpose of your holistic program is to acquire new lifestyle habits, habits that are consistent with whom you really are.

Four Phases of Transformation

As you begin to follow your path of healing the body, mind and Spirit, you will find your journey may progress through a series of phases, each characterized by a subtle shift in both attention and intention.

In the first phase, **Discovery**, you learn how to recognize and distinguish the unique physical body you've created for yourself. You begin to ask questions like, "Where, exactly, are my muscles? What do they do, what do they feel like?" You start to see for yourself if you've created any postural distortions, muscle imbalances or chains of compensation. You also start to notice where Power, Freedom or Flow seem to be missing in your life experience.

The second phase is **Balance**. As you expand your ability to distinguish the masks in your life, you will begin to be able to construct a program to restore the sense of balance in their lives. In this phase, you will learn that a balanced lifestyle operates within what is known as The Wellness Triangle. The three legs of the triangle are 1) Physical Activity, 2) Diet and Nutrition and 3) Stress Management. Each leg of the triangle is equally as important as the other two, so when any leg gets more of your attention, you are actually throwing yourself further out of balance.

The next phase is called **Creativity**. Envision that by this phase you are actually beginning to experience a return to balance, and are conscious of an increase in the sensations of Power, Freedom and Flow. Slowly you will begin to understand that anything is possible. The act of living life is to be an artist, fully involved in "re-creating" yourself. At the same time, however, you will also begin to see that uncovering your own perfection is not the same as being "in control." Instead you'll begin to see, as complexity theory teaches us, that control is a myth. Not to worry, however, for this is actually an opportunity – an opportunity to pay attention to the nuances of the experiences of life. This creates an opening and an opportunity for great creativity.

The fourth phase is the phase of **Synergy**. Here a noticeable shift in the experience of Power, Freedom and Flow is present. Most especially, you will recognize how the process of training has worked, and you will take on being responsible for your own Self, and health. The locus of control has shifted from external to internal. The beauty of this phase is that now body, mind, emotions and Spirit are operating together in harmony and synergy as never before… and the training cycle actually begins again – making new discoveries, distinguishing more places to restore balance, and finding new opportunities for creativity.

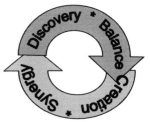

> ### The Holistic Program Recipe
> 1. Look in the Mirror
>   a. 5-season BodyMind test
>   b. Wellness Index
>   c. Postural assessment
> 2. Distinguish your patterns
>   a. Look at the 6 Universal Compensations chart
>   b. What are the Balancing Acts?
>   c. Consult the continua, and choose specific modalities
> 3. Mix your choices according to your BodyMind Season, and serve.

Whipping Up Your Holistic Program

Although holistic workout/diet/stress management plans are as diverse as fingerprints or snowflakes, you can use a basic recipe to prepare your program. Using this formula, every program will have a different flavor and texture, reflecting the not only the ingredients but also the unique individual enjoying it.

Step One: Look in the Mirror

As we saw earlier, the first phase of transformation is Discovery. In this phase, we begin to see with a clearer eye the structures that are in place in your life.

The 5-Season BodyMind Type Test

Take the 5-Season questionnaire to determine your bodymind type. Knowing the characteristics inherent in your temperament will guide you in making choices in your program.

Specifically, you will see things to avoid. Take diets, for example. If you happen to be one of the BodyMind types that are relationship and people-oriented, you should consider that all those diets that are "food-oriented," logical and chemical will just not match your temperament. There's nothing wrong with those diets – you just probably will never be entirely comfortable following them, and you probably won't stick with them very long. And what good will they do you then?

The drives and desires of each Season are most important to know if you want a truly holistic program. In a nutshell: Spring types desire action, and are most inspired by a sense of achievement and power. Summer types want fun, and are most inspired by a sense of spontaneity and freedom. Autumn types want structure, and are motivated by a sense of value and integrity. Indian Summers desire peace and harmony, and are moved by relationship. Finally, Winters want information – or data – and are inspired by the ability to prioritize and strategize.

The Wellness Index Survey

The Wellness Index score will indicate the weakest link in your lifestyle. This principle says that the weakest link is the place of least integrity, the place where your energy of life is leaking out. In addition, the farther apart the weakest link (indicated by your lowest Wellness Index score) is from your strongest link, the more out of balance you are.

One of the important things to remember is that each leg of the Wellness Triangle affects the other two. Poor nutrition, for example, will have an impact on the way your body moves, available energy, strength of the immune system, storage of fat and more. The food you eat also affects your emotions, and may either amplify or quiet the effects of stress. By the same token, your emotional state has an impact on your appetite, your digestion, and your elimination as well – not to mention whether you even feel like being physically active.

The Wellness Index, remember, does not measure the quality of your nutritional choices, nor how relaxing your stress management techniques or functional your exercise regimen. The Wellness Index measures your *awareness* of each of the legs of the Wellness Triangle – in other words, your level of consciousness of each leg. Awareness is another way of saying being connected – and every degree of increased connection among our bodies, minds, emotions and Spirits (and the lifestyle habits that support us) is another step towards balance and the moment-to-moment experience of Power, Freedom and Flow.

Simple Postural Assessment
At first it may seem challenging to identify the specific symptoms of your body's compensations. But with only a little practice these signs will begin to leap out at you. Think of it like learning to speak a foreign language. In the beginning, listening to a conversation in that tongue is incomprehensible. But as your ear improves, words and phrases begin to stand out.

As you learned in the chapter on Kinesiology, divide the body into three basic sections: lower body, middle and upper body. Look for differences from the left side to the right. Look for whatever stands out, and compare it to the imbalances in Tables 1-3.

What do you do if you can't figure it out?

1) Look to the next level – the patterns themselves – and see if the descriptions of the patterns resonate with you in any way.

2) Remember, more than one pattern can be present simultaneously. What we're looking for is the strongest or most dominant pattern. This is another version of the weakest link.

3) Use the website, and if possible send us a digital photo, and we'll work with you to complete your assessment, and help you hone your skills.

Step Two: Distinguish Your Patterns

The masks and compensations are like the beams and scaffolding of a house, holding your body, mind, emotions and Spirit in place. Like any other scaffolding, these patterns and habits hold you in a consistent way of being, effectively restricting your movements, and triggering the same reactions over and over.

Review the 6 Universal Compensations Chart

By now you should be well-acquainted with the idea that what stands between you and the experience of power, freedom and flow are the compensations – the masks – that you have created for yourself in an attempt to create greater functionality. In the body, we see that physical compensations lead to postural distortions, and these distortions in turn lead to further compensations, creating layer upon layer of masks.

Review the Continua

When it comes time to selecting the actual workouts, diets or meditations that fit into your program, you'll of course look to each of the three continua to guide you to selecting your specific workouts, diets or relaxation tools. Yet each "modality" is both a diagnostic assessment tool, and a structure for reshaping the body (and mind and Spirit) and its motions. Every "yoga" is a finger under the mask the gentle hammer that cracks the mask and the microscope that reveals the nature of the mask. The nature of these tools is that they spiral inward, revealing more and providing more access for the body to heal itself.

Look at each continuum through the filter of your specific individual bodymind type at all the options of movement, diet and relaxation. Consider what your real objectives and goals are. At this point, choices may jump out at you yelling, "pick me, pick me!" Or a sense of what fits with your Season may lay quietly in the background of your mind as you also consider the activities that balance the patterns you've distinguished present in your body.

The Balancing Acts

Every compensation pattern represents a pull away from a balanced body, mind and Spirit. But for every force that pulls on us like gravity, dragging us away from balance, there is a possible levitating pattern that will lift us upward to balance once again. We can train these harmonizing patterns into ourselves with new movement practices, and we call these the "Balancing Acts." On the following page is a chart of workouts and exercises that represent a sample of physical balancing acts.

1. Heaviness/Lighten Up
    a. The flipside, or mirror image, of Heaviness is to "lighten up!" Here you would take on movement modalities that allow you to be free and spontaneous, light-hearted and non-achievement oriented. One of the common examples I use is salsa dancing.
2. Stiffness/Loosen Up
    a. The mirror image of Stiffness is to "loosen up." An obvious example of a "loosening up" exercise is hatha yoga – although of course yoga is much more than just stretching.
3. Breaking/Get Connected
    a. On the other side of Breaking – or complete dissociation – is "getting connected." T'ai Chi, ch'i kung, pranayama and other styles of meditation all methods of bringing the pieces of the self back together.
4. Lightness/Pay Attention
    a. While Breaking is complete dissociation, Lightness is merely on the way there. When lightness is the pattern, I recommend exercises that train you to really "pay attention." For example, Systematic T.O.U.C.H. Training – or STT – is a system that uses hands on coaching to help you really get in touch with your muscles as you move.
5. Misdirection/Return to the Center
    a. Misdirection reflects a special kind of disconnection – disconnection from the center. The literal center of the body is the thoracic core, so the balance of misdirection is exercise for the "Core" – the abs and lower back.
6. Monotony/Create Variety
    a. Finally, the balance of Monotony – the tendency to move and act in the same way over and over again – is to seek variety. One of the most innovative workouts I've seen is called Nia (Neuromuscular Integrative Action). Nia uses free-flowing and spontaneous moves derived from dance, martial arts and yoga. Every class is unique, and the experience of Nia is truly one of infinite variety.

Step Three: Mix your choices according to your BodyMind Season, and serve.

Once you have determined your BodyMind type and the weakest leg of your Wellness Triangle, taken a look at the continua and the balancing acts, it's time to mix together all of the ingredients into a program for yourself. In one sense this is the most difficult part, for it comes down to the actual *doing* if one wants to truly break up the old patterns and replace them with the new.

Yet although the doing must be consistent, holistic programs won't feel forced or imposed. This is because the programs are served up according to each individual's BodyMind Season, and reflects how they themselves view the world. To give you a taste of this, I've included in this chapter six six-week sample programs – three programs each for Summers and Indian Summers. In fact, you can even use these sample programs as your own, filling in the elements appropriate to you.

Cooking Tip: Each BodyMind Season processes the world in a unique manner. Their bodies, minds and emotions handle the flow of information and the stimulus of new sensations in different ways. Consequently each different Season should train their new patterns in a specific rhythm, with a specific level of intensity.

Spring types should cook up a program in which they practice four days/week with a high challenge level. Summer types, on the other hand do better when they practice three to four days/week, doing something different every day. Indian Summer types should be active a lot – five to seven days/week, and I recommend they do it with a friend or group of friends. Autumn types should only work out three to four days/week, progressing along a detailed linear menu of activities. Finally, Winters should train four to six days/week, and re-evaluate their program every six months.

Sample Six-Week Programs -- Phase One: Discovery.

Objectives: To discover and catalog symptoms, compensations and masks.

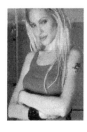

- **Summer**
  - Psycho-physio profile: The Free Spirit; small-medium meso-morph. Lean dancer's body; will try new, fun things.
  - Intrinsic Motivator: Spontaneity
  - Inner Destabilizer: Giving too much
  - Reaction: Emotional burnout/mood swings
  - Compatible Workouts: Hatha yoga, low-impact aerobics, dance, jazzercise, Nia, circuit-training
  - **Regimen: 3-4 days/wk – something different @ day**

1. Summer → variety and fun = fulfillment
   a. Stress Management as weak leg
      i. Week One
         1. Relaxation Training, appropriate to observed core dynamic.
         2. Important: start a diary of the compensations and dynamics you observe
         3. Create new structures for independent training (creating new patterns).
         4. Create the context for variety and spontaneity.
      ii. Week Two
         1. Relaxation Training, appropriate to observed core dynamic.
         2. Reinforcing techniques, adding new to program.
         3. Be creative, and draw a picture of your practice on a chart
      iii. Week Three
         1. Exercise Training, *appropriate to observed core dynamic.*

                2. Focus on something fun and moderately challenging.
                3. Add to your picture, logging your progress.
            iv. Week Four
                1. Relaxation Training, appropriate to observed core dynamic.
                2. Add to your picture, logging your progress.
                3. Give client Diet Diary to fill out for following week.
            v. Week Five
                1. Diet Training, appropriate to observed core dynamic.
                2. Focus on source of major observed compensations (usually relationship to food).
                3. Order metabolic testing kit.
                4. Add to your picture, logging your progress.
            vi. Week Six
                1. Relaxation Training, appropriate to observed core dynamic.
                2. Add to your picture, logging your progress.
                3. Take new assessments to measure degree of reduction of major compensations.
                4. Review your progress chart and imagine the next phase.
    b. Diet as weak leg
        i. Week One
            1. Diet Training, appropriate to observed core dynamic.
            2. Important: clearly document observed compensations and dynamics
            3. Create new structures for independent training (creating new patterns).
            4. Create the context for variety and spontaneity.
            5. Start your Diet Diary.
            6. Order metabolic testing kit.

ii. Week Two
   1. Diet Training, appropriate to observed core dynamic.
   2. Reinforcing techniques, adding new to program.
   3. Add to your picture, logging your progress.
iii. Week Three
   1. Exercise Training, appropriate to observed core dynamic.
   2. Focus on something fun and moderately challenging.
   3. Add to your picture, logging your progress.
iv. Week Four
   1. Diet Training, appropriate to observed core dynamic.
   2. Reinforcing techniques, adding new to program.
   3. Add to your picture, logging your progress.
v. Week Five
   1. Relaxation Training, appropriate to observed core dynamic.
   2. Suggestion: Guided Visualization
vi. Week Six
   1. Diet Training, appropriate to observed core dynamic.
   2. Add to your picture, logging your progress.
   3. Take new assessments to measure degree of reduction of major compensations.
   4. Review your progress chart and discuss look ahead to the next phase.

c. Physical Activity as weak leg
   i. Week One
      1. Exercise Training, appropriate to observed core dynamic.

2. Important: clearly document observed compensations and dynamics
3. Create new structures for independent training (creating new patterns).
4. Create the context for variety and spontaneity.

ii. Week Two
   1. Exercise Training, appropriate to observed core dynamic.
   2. Reinforcing techniques, adding new to program.
   3. Add to your picture, logging your progress.

iii. Week Three
   1. Diet Training, appropriate to observed core dynamic.
   2. Focus on source of major observed compensations (usually relationship to food).
   3. Order metabolic testing kit.
   4. Add to your picture, logging your progress.

iv. Week Four
   1. Exercise Training, appropriate to observed core dynamic.
   2. Reinforcing techniques, adding new to program.
   3. Add to your picture, logging your progress.

v. Week Five
   1. Relaxation Training, appropriate to observed core dynamic.
   2. Suggestion: Guided Visualization

vi. Week Six
   1. Exercise Training, appropriate to observed core dynamic.
   2. Add to your picture, logging your progress.
   3. Take new assessments to measure degree of reduction of major compensations.
   4. Add to your picture, logging your progress.

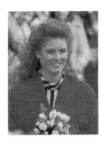

- Indian Summer
- Psycho-physio profile: The Nurturing Spirit; systemic thinkers; endomorph, slower metabolism, need to be early risers
- Intrinsic Motivator: Relationship
- Inner Destabilizer: Lethargy
- Reaction: Couch potato
- Compatible Workouts: Walking, jazzercise, T'ai Chi Ch'uan, swimming, tennis, cycling, circuit training
- **Regimen: 5-7 days/week with a partner**

2. Indian Summer → Relationship and partnership = fulfillment
   a. Stress Management as weak leg
      i. Week One
         1. Relaxation Training, appropriate to observed core dynamic.
         2. Important: clearly document observed compensations and dynamics
         3. Create new structures for independent training (creating new patterns).
         4. Create the context for relatedness and partnership.
      ii. Week Two
         1. Relaxation Training, appropriate to observed core dynamic.
         2. Reinforcing techniques, adding new to program.
         3. Keep track of your practice on a chart.
      iii. Week Three
         1. Exercise Training, appropriate to observed core dynamic.
         2. Focus on core training and stability.
      iv. Week Four
         1. Relaxation Training, appropriate to observed core dynamic.

                2. Reinforcing techniques, adding new to program.
                3. Keep track of your practice on a chart.
            v. Week Five
                1. Diet Training, appropriate to observed core dynamic.
                2. Focus on source of major observed compensations (usually relationship to food).
                3. Order metabolic testing kit.
                4. Keep track of your practice on a chart.
            vi. Week Six
                1. Relaxation Training, appropriate to observed core dynamic.
                2. Trainer logs client's practice on chart (with client).
                3. Take new assessments to measure degree of reduction of major compensations.
                4. Keep track of your practice on a chart.

    b. Diet as weak leg Diet as weak leg
        i. Week One
            1. Diet Training, appropriate to observed core dynamic.
            2. Important: clearly document observed compensations and dynamics
            3. Create new structures for independent training (creating new patterns).
            4. Create the context for relatedness and partnership.
            5. Start a Diet Diary.
            6. Order metabolic testing kit.
        ii. Week Two
            1. Diet Training, appropriate to observed core dynamic.

        2. Reinforcing techniques, adding new to program.

        3. Keep track of your practice on a chart.

   iii. Week Three

        1. Exercise Training, appropriate to observed core dynamic.

        2. Focus on something fun and moderately challenging.

        3. Keep track of your practice on a chart.

   iv. Week Four

        1. Diet Training, appropriate to observed core dynamic.

        2. Reinforcing techniques, adding new to program.

        3. Keep track of your practice on a chart.

   v. Week Five

        1. Relaxation Training, appropriate to observed core dynamic.

        2. Suggestion: Guided Visualization

   vi. Week Six

        1. Diet Training, appropriate to observed core dynamic.

        2. Keep track of your practice on a chart.

        3. Take new assessments to measure degree of reduction of major compensations.

        4. Review client's progress chart together and discuss next phase.

c. Physical Activity as weak leg

   i. Week One

        1. Exercise Training, appropriate to observed core dynamic.

        2. Important: clearly document observed compensations and dynamics

        3. Create new structures for independent training (creating new patterns).

4. Create the context for variety and spontaneity.

ii. Week Two
   1. Exercise Training, appropriate to observed core dynamic.
   2. Reinforcing techniques, adding new to program.
   3. Keep track of your practice on a chart.

iii. Week Three
   1. Diet Training, appropriate to observed core dynamic.
   2. Focus on source of major observed compensations (usually relationship to food).
   3. Order metabolic testing kit.
   4. Keep track of your practice on a chart.

iv. Week Four
   1. Exercise Training, appropriate to observed core dynamic.
   2. Reinforcing techniques, adding new to program.
   3. Keep track of your practice on a chart.

v. Week Five
   1. Relaxation Training, appropriate to observed core dynamic.
   2. Suggestion: Guided Visualization

vi. Week Six
   1. Exercise Training, appropriate to observed core dynamic.
   2. Keep track of your practice on a chart.
   3. Take new assessments to measure degree of reduction of major compensations.
   4. Review client's progress chart together and discuss next phase.

A Final Thought

When I was 21 I imagined that the purpose of earthly life was to change, to evolve, to "become." The universe, and all the things in it, is constantly changing shape, form and function. This is called evolution, a constant guiding principle of our cosmos.

Whatever we evolve into, I believed, is up to us. I believed the idea that we are the authors of our own lives, the directors of our own movies. A human life was about becoming whatever we want to be. The tragedy of human existence was that we settle for too little, and didn't have enough -- faith? gumption? energy? will power? -- to "go for it" in life. The great tragedy of human history was that we had stayed "merely human" for too long.

Of course, I knew that the process of personal evolution wasn't easy. There are a thousand unseen forces constantly at work to influence and shape our minds, bodies and spirits. Like hurricane force winds, they blow us first this way and then that way, until the ship of our lives has blown so far off course that it seems easier never to have had a destination in the first place. We wind up "evolving by accident," instead of "becoming on purpose."

"They key to becoming on purpose," I wrote in my journal, "is self-control. It is the rudder to the ship of life which allows us to follow the star charts of our desires, steering through the hurricanes of chance." In order to evolve in a purposeful, meaningful way, we first have to develop the skills of self-discipline and self-control. Self-discipline is what gives us the ability to make better choices at the crossroads of life. Making better choices is what keeps us on the path towards our goals, and insures that we wind up becoming the people we want to be.

Before we can claim the power of self-control, we have to know the person we are now. Prerequisite to the skill of self-discipline is the skill of self-awareness. Knowing where you are -- and more importantly, who you are -- is the first step toward the goal of conscious evolution.

Self-control is much different from being self-controlling, in the negative or pathological sense. Obviously, it's not healthy to repress or deny your thoughts and emotions, which is how we often think of "control." "Control," writes Dr. Ken Pelletier, " is a dynamic, ongoing, lifelong process that involves an interplay among rational thought, intuition, conviction and external circumstances... It is not a fixed, static end-point."

Yet before we can exert this kind of self-control, we must become more fully aware of what our actions, thoughts and feelings actually are. Evolution, personal growth and transformation (all names for the same thing) take place in every domain: physical, mental, emotional and Spiritual. Self-discovery takes place on every level as well. But of all our domains, the physical seems to be the most easily discovered. The physical realm is our primary dimension. It is the dimension we can actually see and feel and touch. We can weigh and measure the changes that take place there, which gives us more confidence in the growth process, and the lessons we learn on this level can be translated into lessons about the other levels.

At age 21 I knew that life was a three-stage process, progressing from self-awareness to self-discipline, and finally to conscious change. This is the Warriors Path, the "path of impeccability," as Carlos Casteneda's teacher calls it: to tread each step in your life carefully, mindfully, and with purpose.

Now I am 40, and everything seems different. I still believe in evolution, but now I call it "transformation," and I wonder if we don't evolve from warriors when we are 21 into poets when we are 40. As I write this book about the Holistic approach, I envision it as a way to live poetically, not militantly. You don't have to be perfectly integrated to be soulful; you just have to be willing to be. Willing to *be*. Natalie Goldberg, in her beautiful little book *Wild Mind*, reminds us that the truths you have digested don't have to be paraded about or shouted out; they just float inside of you, communicating silently. "For instance," writes Goldberg, "in a good vegetable soup the onion is not constantly sticking its head up for extra attention and yelling, 'I'm the onion! I'm the onion!' Instead, it is contributing with the other vegetables to the good flavor of the soup."

Genesis

The gift of these final thoughts is *possibility*. You have read the book. What's next? Your health and happiness is only the beginning. Open this gift, and I hope to hear you say, "What can I give back to the world?"

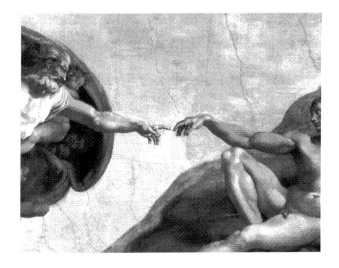

Healing the Soul of the World

> *"What a piece of work is man! How noble in reason! how infinite in faculties! in form and moving, how express and admirable! in action how like an angel! in apprehension, how like a god!"* Hamlet, Act II

We began this book together with the story of the Emperor's wise doctor. He was, as you remember, famous for his ability to heal. All the people in his village, and eventually across his entire province, knew of his miraculous talent for curing any kind of illness or injury. What he did for all the people in his village was literally to "put them back together." Healing is a reconnection – a making whole – of things torn apart. Specifically, healing is the restoration of a feeling, of an experience of life – an experience of being perfect and complete.

Healing is also the path to happiness – the kind of complete fulfillment expressed by the ancient Greek concept of eudaemonia, the full exercise of the soul's powers. The road to happiness lies in discovering the inner dynamic that is running all the engines of your life. In the emotional sensation/perception cycle, when you can distinguish that you have made up the stories (perceptions) that "explain" your emotional reactions to life's events (sensation), then you have the power to choose stories that empower and affirm you.

Recently, one of my clients and I were on a walk together, talking about having a point of view in life. I commented that points of view weren't necessarily true or false, they're literally just where you look out from – and that gives you what you see. "For instance," I said, "I'm just a glass half-full rather than a glass half-empty kind of guy."

"Oh no," she said. "You are most definitely *not* a glass half-full kind of guy."

"I'm not?"

"No! You're a glass FULL kind of guy!"

Life doesn't part around me like the Red Sea did for Moses. I still get stuck in traffic, have to pay taxes and get stranded in airports from time to time. But I have chosen to interpret life's events in soulful and Spiritual ways, rather than only mundane and material ways.

One of the effects of the Holistic approach is an awakening to a *soulful* experience of life, where soul is the word I would give to the conscious awareness of being perfect and complete. Here life occurs as the miraculous interweaving of body, thoughts, emotions and Spirit, and power, freedom and flow course through our lives every minute of every day

Soul, in a way, is nothing more or less than *authenticity*. We can speak of authenticity as acting, speaking, thinking, and feeling in alignment with our fundamental reality – namely, that we are absolutely perfect. Soul, in other words, is an experience of relative authenticity in our lives. We are happiest when we are the most soulful, the most authentic and the most connected with ourselves on all levels.

On the other hand, inauthentic behavior is to act (and/or believe) as other than we are. It is, in the words of the existentialists, a self-lie. To be kind, our self-lies are mostly unintentional. The world around us occurs continuously as "something is wrong" or "something is missing." In that case, of course we would reasonably behave as though there *is* something wrong with us, something wrong with the world, something missing in our lives or in our relationships. But inauthentic attitudes and behaviors, though perhaps unconscious, don't go unnoticed. The very thought that something is wrong or missing itself seems wrong or incomplete. Unsatisfactory. It occurs as a decline in the quality of our experience of life – a *loss* of soul.

But remember, the wise healer considered his brother to be the greater doctor. The brother taught all his villagers to live so that they never got disconnected from soul in the first place. His philosophy was that soul is elusive when you try to get at it through Conventional fix-it approaches. Much better, he seemed to say, to preserve the connection between body, mind, emotions, soul and Spirit than to try to restore the connection when it is lost. That kind of approach is a Holistic one. It did not focus on any one aspect of our Selves, nor on any one leg of the wellness triangle. In fact, the Holistic approach of the wise doctor's brother ties together threads of life often ignored entirely by Conventional approaches.

"Soul," writes Thomas Moore, "lies midway between understanding and unconsciousness, and its instrument is neither the mind nor the body, but imagination." The imagination is one of the four essential characteristics of Classical Mind/Body Exercise. The other three are spinal alignment, breathing and relaxation. When all four are combined, magic happens, and the qi – the inner energy of life, flows like a river in the body. Leave one or more of the four ingredients out, and the river slows to a trickle.

The imagination, or the faculty of visualization, is called in Chinese the *I* (pronounced "Eee"), which translates as the "mind-intent." One of the most famous and fundamental T'ai Chi aphorisms is, *I dao, qi dao* which means, "The mind arrives and then the qi arrives." Where the mind goes, the qi follows. Said another way, where you send your imagination and will, the energy of your life will go there.

If the energy of our imagination goes continually towards "something is wrong with me – I'm broken and I need to be fixed or improved," then that is where the energy of our lives will go. To be human is to have the complete package – body, mind, emotions and Spirit. Without any of these elements, we wouldn't be human beings. And yet, dissociating from those parts of life we find difficult, frightening or ugly is something we do all the time. Is it any wonder so many of us are chronically ill or in pain, that we die too young, before living out the fullness of our possible lifespan, or that we suffer the aches and agonies of life's emotional disappointments that are so frequently part of the human experience?

By the way, I am not someone who believes that suffering is necessary for growth and wisdom. That, to me, is the voice of resignation and cynicism. I wonder what other realms of experience we could break through if we didn't spend so much time in suffering. If we but direct our will power to the image of ourselves as perfect, whole and complete, then *that* is the direction our qi will flow.

> *"Man... finds identity in the extent to which he commits himself to something beyond himself, to a cause greater than himself."* -- Viktor Frankl

Another place where soul shows up is in your contribution to community. Moore says, "Relatedness is a signal of the soul." As I wrote in the beginning of Chapter I, I believe that when every person in the world has the opportunity for health and freedom from suffering, then war will disappear, as will poverty, prejudice and violence. Creating your own health heals the planet – *your* piece of the planet, anyway. "No man is an island," John Donne wrote. "Every man's death diminishes me, because I am involved in Mankind." If Donne had lived today, he might have also written "every man or woman's health also heals me."

Every day I thank God for the privilege of doing the work I do. Every person I meet reminds me of the incredible nobility of the human Spirit, and the terrible beauty of the human experience. I am thinking about the 20 year-old girl suffering from severe back pain who had never heard the words, "Your back may be in pain, but there's nothing wrong with *you.*" I remember the man who asked me what I would say to someone who had terminal cancer. Would I still say he was perfect? We talked about the body as metaphor, about how the body sometimes has to get our attention if we have ignored it too long. "You know, you're right," he said. "It wasn't until about five years ago that I even knew I had a body. Up until then I thought it was a car." He thought for a moment, and then said, "I guess in my case my body felt so ignored it had to grab me and slam me to the ground."

As I travel around the world, lecturing and leading seminars, over and over the people I meet thank me for being committed to the health and happiness of others, and they ask me how they can also be a contribution. So I started two twin ventures, The Wellness Evolution website, and the Zenergy Neighborhood Wellness Centers™. In these two projects I have planted what I hope are the seeds of global community, and I am extending an invitation for everyone I meet, or who reads this book, to see if there is a place here for you to get involved.

The idea behind Zenergy™ is to create "neighborhood-based" wellness centers. No longer will you have to go to the gym, or to the mall, or to a professional building somewhere to learn the best way to move your body, manage your stress or eat for health. Instead, wellness will be right next-door, around the corner, or up the street in your own neighborhood. What will this give us? A shift toward a culture in which wellness is part of your natural local environment, and in which everyone at the most grass roots level is empowered to make informed, healthy lifestyle choices.

The Zenergy Wellness Center™ is designed to be in a house – like *your* house. The men and women who run the Center work primarily one-on-one with clients or with some small group classes (3-4 people). What they offer is professional wellness coaching along the three legs of the Wellness Triangle: physical activity, stress management and nutrition. There will be space in this house for movement and activity, of course. There will also be quiet rooms for reflection and meditation, and conversations between the clients and their coaches. And there will be a kitchen, where people can learn not only the technical side of good nutrition, but they can learn how to actually cook delicious healthy meals!

The other project I'm involved with is a virtual on-line community called The Wellness Evolution. A significant part of my travel schedule is dedicated to leading intensive extended seminars certifying fitness professionals in a new designation called the Mind/Body Personal Trainer. Once I started holding the certifications, it became apparent that there was an opportunity to invite people all over the world to form a community, the purpose of which was to support each other in the teaching of holistic health. I was inspired to call this group *The Wellness Evolution*, since what we're up to represents the future of the fitness and health care industry, including but transcending all the practices we've been using up until now. In community, I feel, we can be unstoppable, generous contributors to the vision of global health.

The opportunity of the Wellness Evolution is to be a part of a movement to expand what is possible in fitness, wellness and health. Imagine the difference it would make if there were simply a new conversation occurring around the world about the hows and whys of our industry's philosophy and best practices. What we're saying is that current practices do not effectively impact enough people.

Our specific objectives are to establish a global community of certified Mind/body personal trainers, holistic health practitioners and other interested persons, engaged in an on-going conversation about expanding what is possible in the realm of fitness, wellness and health, with 10,000 members by December 31, 2003; and to organize an international conference that will convene in February 2004.

If you are inspired by either of these two projects, I invite you to contact us through our website: www.thewellnessevolution.com. I look forward to hearing from you!

Namaste

One of the most popular Holistic practices these days is hatha yoga, and while not all yoga practice is Holistic, and certainly the Holistic approach is not synonymous with doing yoga, yoga does serve as a beautiful metaphor for what the Holistic approach offers. The word yoga means "the yoke" -- the device that connects part A (your senses) to part B (the experience of your health and happiness). The Holistic approach is on the one hand nothing more than a device, a key to opening the doorway to an experience of power, freedom and flow. On the other hand, the Holistic approach is itself a life-affirming philosophy and lifestyle that is meant to heal the body and feed the soul.

Hatha yoga has a life-affirming philosophy as well, and even expresses that philosophy in the language of its practice. Traditional yoga classes usually end with the teacher and students placing their hands together in front of their hearts in a prayer position, and saying to each other, "Namaste." Namaste is a sanskrit word, a derivative of the word that means to salute, to acknowledge... to recognize. Specifically, this single word, exchanged between teacher and student, means, "I see inside you the beautiful light of your Spirit, and I salute it."

The last pose of every yoga practice is Savasana, the Corpse Pose. But it's not a corpse as in being dead and lifeless. It's a corpse in the sense of ultimate rest and renewal. And what is on the other side of death, anyway? According to yogic tradition, the other side of death is rebirth. For an hour or so of a hatha yoga practice, the yogi (or yogin) stretches, twists and flexes his or her body, transforming it physically cell by cell, and preparing it for the rigors of meditation. Then the yogi lays quietly, letting go of all the effort and concentration of the previous hour. And when he or she finally awakens, they are metaphorically reborn, ready to walk out into life with new eyes, a new body, and a new heart and soul.

At the end of every yoga class, as my students are coming out of Savasana, I tell them this: Every time you practice yoga, it gets easier. It gets easier to remember the names of all the postures, and how to make those particular shapes with your body. It gets easier to remember how and when to breathe, and how to relax into the poses so that they are as comfortable as an old familiar chair. But most of all, it gets easier to remember the most fundamental philosophy that is at the heart of yoga practice – that right now, in this very moment, *you are absolutely perfect*. And you don't need to go anywhere or do anything to get more perfect than you already are. All you need to do is part the curtain, or clear away the mist, that covers up your appreciation for how perfect you are. And every time you practice, it gets just a little bit easier to do that. I wish you health, wealth and harmony. Namaste…

Made in the USA